T0275894

FAST FACTS FOR WOUND CARE NURSING

Practical Wound Management in a Nutshell

Zelia Ann Kifer, RN, BSN, CWS

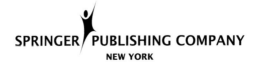

SPRINGER PUBLISHING COMPANY

NEW YORK

Copyright © 2012 Springer Publishing Company, LLC

Springer Publishing Company, LLC
11 West 42nd Street
New York, NY 10036
www.springerpub.com

Acquisitions Editor: Margaret Zuccarini
Composition: Newgen Imaging

ISBN: 978-0-8261-0775-6
E-book ISBN: 978-0-8261-0776-3

11 12 13 / 5 4 3 2 1

The author and the publisher of this Work have made every effort to use sources believed to be reliable to provide information that is accurate and compatible with the standards generally accepted at the time of publication. The author and publisher shall not be liable for any special, consequential, or exemplary damages resulting, in whole or in part, from the readers' use of, or reliance on, the information contained in this book. The publisher has no responsibility for the persistence or accuracy of URLs for external or third-party Internet Web sites referred to in this publication and does not guarantee that any content on such Web sites is, or will remain, accurate or appropriate.

Library of Congress Cataloging-in-Publication Data

Kifer, Zelia Ann.
   Fast facts for wound care nursing : practical wound management in a
nutshell / Zelia Ann Kifer.
      p. ; cm.
   Includes bibliographical references and index.
   ISBN 978-0-8261-0775-6 (alk. paper) — ISBN 978-0-8261-0776-3 (e-book)
   I. Title.
   [DNLM: 1. Wound Healing—Handbooks. 2. Wounds and
Injuries—nursing—Handbooks. WO 39]
      617.1—dc23   2011035185

Special discounts on bulk quantities of our books are available to corporations, professional associations, pharmaceutical companies, health care organizations, and other qualifying groups.

If you are interested in a custom book, including chapters from more than one of our titles, we can provide that service as well.

For details, please contact:
Special Sales Department, Springer Publishing Company, LLC
11 West 42nd Street, 15th Floor, New York, NY 10036-8002
Phone: 877-687-7476 or 212-431-4370; Fax: 212-941-7842
Email: sales@springerpub.com

Printed in the United States of America by Bang Printing

I dedicate this book to my clinical friends, colleagues, and patients who "parted the Red Sea" of clinical experiences and to my husband who financially "walked on water" so I could write this book.

Zelia Ann Kifer, RN, BSN, CWS, served as a Advanced Wound and Skin Care Specialist (AWSCS) for Medline Industries, Inc. Medline is a fast-growing distributor of medical and surgical supplies in the United States, servicing more than 250 hospitals and offering a comprehensive array of consulting and management services, including on-staff clinicians. Zelia was one of the top-ranking AWSCS for Medline, helping to implement training for new wound care representatives in the field, and establish Wound and Skin Care Protocols and Guidelines for a variety of hospital systems, long-term acute care facilities (LTAC's) and nursing homes. In addition, she served nationally and internationally as Medline's Burn Care Specialist and presented continuing education (CE) courses on various topics in burn, wound, and skin care. She is a Certified Wound Specialist (CWS), a member of Sigma Theta Tau International and of the WOCN.

As a board-certified Advanced Burn Specialist (ABS), Zelia worked as a ICU Burn Nurse, and then as the charge nurse responsible for the outpatient burn clinic and tank room, at The Alexander Burn Center in Tulsa, Oklahoma, from 1996–2000.

Zelia has given many seminars and presentations across the United States, and has conducted on-site in-services and training for clinical staff of all levels, educating OR, ICU, Peds/NICU, Oncology, Cardiac, and Med-Surg nurses. She is the author of *Sculpting the Heart of a Nurse—A Book to Energize the Novice, Rejuvenate the Exhausted and Challenge the Average.* She helped establish The Tulsa Medical Mission Team and the Medical Mission Room that provides burn care in Honduras. During her recent 2010 Annual Medical Mission visit, the team mentored residents and nurses through 15 successful burn surgeries.

Contents

Section III—Wound Care Treatment and Protocols

Section IV—Legal Aspects and Regulations

Foreword

Wound healing has been a lifelong fascination for me. At a very young age, a messenger at the door informed me that my mom had been hurt while picking apricots in a neighbors orchard. That I was an 8 year old left to look after younger siblings was not unusual: it was a time when parents could go out and do chores while leaving an older child to look after the younger siblings, a time when neighbors acted like parents, a time when it didn't seem strange when a family friend came in to make us sandwiches as a stand-in for our mom. All day we waited for mom to come home to start dinner, and when she hadn't by the time dad pulled in from work, we were pretty sure something bad had happened. Mom only came home for a few weeks over the next year and a half, while doctors and nurses battled to repair a compound fracture of her lower leg. Although the bones finally mended well enough so that she eventually could walk again, the soft tissue injury did not. Little did we know that our family would begin an 18 year witness of my mom's non-healing wound.

Looking back, I marvel at how that injury, brought on by a misplaced ladder, influenced my career path. The injury provided a lesson about resilience of the patient and acceptance by a family. Eventually, mom was able to function a lot like a normal mom: sending us to school, making sure we had clean clothes, playing baseball, preparing dinners. She accomplished all this in spite of her injured leg, which was measurably shorter than her other leg and also had a fairly decent-sized hole in it. When I watched her change the dressing I would catch a glimpse of the yellow-white bone deep at the base of the wound, and wonder why that wound didn't seem to hurt her and why it didn't heal like my scrapes and cuts did. Throughout high school and my early university years I heard various answers to my wound healing questions, but most of them communicated a central theme: infection! Infection, likewise, seemed to point me in the direction of microbiology as a major, and a career goal of finding a way to resolve infection so that the wound would heal.

Perhaps better drugs, improved clinical interventions, or maybe simply cessation of smoking resulted in a final closure of her wound after 18 years. I continued to teach and conduct research in microbiology and immunology, until my chance involvement in a research project that developed a sophisticated polymer containing properties supporting the creation of an optimal condition to promote wound healing. I was so intrigued with the benefits that the material could lend to wound healing that I left the university to dedicate my career to exploring tools and strategies for the management of the non-healing wound.

Until recently, wound healing largely has been an art, probably with prehistoric beginnings. It has long been recognized that almost any wound would heal if infection didn't kill the patient first—but that adage applied to 'most' wounds, not those few exceptional wounds that wouldn't heal. Those non-healing wounds weren't talked about much. Over a career of attempting to improve the tools for wound care, I have observed perhaps a thousand non-healing wounds. I have been intrigued at how many patients have become resigned to "living" with their wound. One lady lived with a venous stasis ulcer for over 32 years. It was just a "little problem...." she said she "lived with." Much like my mom's 18 year saga with the non-healing hole in her leg, it was just part of the family.

Professional wound care statistics for the numbers of chronic non-healing wounds in the United States are surely an under-estimation of the actual number in our communities. Coping with the wound is the norm rather than an exception; partly ingrained from unsatisfactory outcomes of a failed prior intervention. Clinicians often "discover" a wound, rather that respond to one as a primary complaint for a visit.

These patients should be encouraged to try new wound care strategies, because wound care has come a long way in the past 30 years. Some medical schools are beginning to offer training in the subject, which perhaps shows there is increased confidence that intervention in non-healing wounds can make a difference. I have been intrigued at the explosion in new technologies that have been cleared for use in the clinical environment. These have ranged from sophisticated materials for controlling and optimizing conditions for healing in the wounds; antimicrobial wound dressings to combat microbial colonization and infection; biological materials that act by competing for bad-news enzymes that chew up healthy tissues; and extremely complex artificial tissues for closure of wounds. In addition there have been major leaps in understanding of the reasons why some wounds don't heal, including overproduction of matrix metalloproteases, decreased perfusion, poor oxygenation, and lack of nutrition.

We can expect that research and innovation will deliver continuing improvements in the range and effectiveness of tools for combating non-healing wounds, including topical delivery of nutrition and oxygen and better methods of controlling bioburdens in wounds. Clinicians will have access to sophisticated instrumentation that will aid healing and perhaps enable the monitoring of success in healing.

It should be taken as a fact that these developments will occur. However in the trenches it will still be people: The clinicians that take care of these wounds; the nurses and doctors that map out the strategies for closing these defects; the wound care specialists who monitor the successes and failures of those strategies; the people that have to make hard decisions and argue with payers to change modalities.

Wound care is arguably the single most difficult topic in medicine. It has no defined solution akin to insulin for the diabetic. It has no easy strategy that covers all wounds. Even with the best and newest of products, there are no easy answers. That is why it is so important for those that have successes to share their experiences with others. Sometimes that can be done one on one, but that isn't tremendously efficient in reaching the ever increasing numbers of clinicians now specializing in wound care. That is why we are so tremendously blessed when one of them, like Zelia, will carve out time to capture a career of experiences in text so that it can be shared with others. We are indebted to her for making this important contribution to the clinicians armament for dealing with the difficult-to-heal wounds of their patients.

Bruce Gibbins, PhD
Founder, Chief Technical Officer and
Chairman of the Board
AcryMed, Inc.
Former faculty at the University of
Otago Medical School

Preface

"Wounds"—What a broad term?! *The Original Roget's International Thesaurus* gives all of the following terms for "wounds": trauma, injury, hurt, lesion, cut, incision, scratch, gash, puncture, stab, laceration, mutilation, abrasion, scuff, scrape, chafe, slash, burn, scald, fracture, bruise, inflamed, gangrene, necrosis, disease, sick, ill, suffer, death. If Roget were a nurse looking at a wound for the first time, he wouldn't stop with just a simple surface term. In a split second, he would send all that information to his mental search engine for processing. His simple surface term, *abrasion,* would generate more sensory input such as: classifications—common, complex, or atypical, chronic or acute; bioburden—clean, dirty, infected, and so on. Before heaving a big sigh, he might have contemplated nutrition and pain management. After all this was sufficiently processed, another broad term would surface. "I need a *remedy.*" Roget's brain interface system would go into overdrive, bouncing from neuron to neuron as more definitions came to mind, such as: relief, help, restorative, medicine, drug, soothing, debridement, salve, antibiotics, poultices, bandage, healing, curative, restorative, palliative, protective ... oh, and coming up for air ... preventive. Whew!

Before your brain dendrites recoil: I am a certified wound care specialist and my goal is to simplify the wound care process for you. The wound care information in this book was written in the *Fast Facts* format to give you, the reader, user-friendly ease of access when needing specific answers regarding the scope of wound care. This book is friendly and non-intimidating, making it a "must read" for the nursing student or the nurse with a passion for pursuing the specialty of wound care.

We've come a long way since the old "barber pole" days and wet-to-dry dressings. Just knowing there are over 150 wound care companies that provide over 1,000 wound care products boggles even the specialized nurse's mind. Not only has the treatment for wounds become complex, but so have the legal aspects of wound care. It is no surprise that wound care has grown into its own specialty. Specialization? Simplification. This book will cut out the wordy textbook style and simplify and re-enforce knowledge for the nurse dedicated to providing ideal wound care in the most cost-efficient way possible. This book will also be an ideal reference guide no matter your level of wound care interest, educational preparation, or even years of work experience. The book is designed to be an easy read, bullet pointed with practical information.

Each chapter includes a brief introduction and a feature entitled "Fast Facts in a Nutshell" that provides insight to important wound care principles for your consideration. I encourage you to take note and enjoy your wound care discoveries.

Acknowledgments

This book is a cooperative effort based on the ideals of professionals across the spectrum of wound care, so my attempts to acknowledge all the contributions will essentially fall short. To all the nurses who have crossed my clinical path, either in the working trenches or during facilitated in-services: I acknowledge and thank you for your spirit, shared memories, and cherished friendships. Your passion encourages me profoundly!

I thank God for channeling my faith and providing opportunity through many epiphanies during my nursing journey that have led to the origin of this book. All my endeavors would be nothing without His wisdom, love, and guidance. I also thank my husband, Roger Kifer, for his devotion and unconditional love. He is truly a man among men for the way he sacrificed his time and provided me the working freedom I needed to complete this project. Thank you from the bottom of my heart. To my family, especially Ruth and Mom, who tag-teamed me by taking up the slack and helping me with all my other responsibilities (and projects): My unending gratitude to you all! I owe a huge debt of gratitude to Gary Williams, MD and Murray Katcher, MD at the Department of Pediatrics of The University of Wisconsin, Madison for permission to reprint their "Primary Care Dermatology Module Nomenclature of Skin Lesions."

I would also like to thank my Publisher, Margaret Zuccarini, Springer Publishing Company, and all the individuals who reviewed the manuscript for accuracy. Your advice, support, and confidence helped make this book possible.

And last (but not least): I would like to thank *you*, the reader, for your passion in wound care. My intent is that this book be a benefit to you, helping you to facilitate ideal wound care to every one of your uniquely special patients and their distinctive, individual wounds.

Thank you all ever so much!

Assessment, Measurement, and Documentation

Attacking the Basics: Know what Fuels a Wound and Understand the Outcome Goal

INTRODUCTION

Simply put, there are three components that control the existence and outcome of a wound:

1. The wound environment (patient).
2. The nurse (caretaker).
3. The dressing (manufacture).

Each of these components plays a key role in whether or not an acceptable or positive outcome is achieved. Also, each of these components influences the desired timeframe of a realistic outcome. You must develop your own approach to wound care. As Confucius said, "By nature, men are nearly alike; by practice, they get to be wide apart." In essence, the same is true of wounds and dressings: No two wounds or dressings are exactly alike. This chapter will help you understand how to start your approach for best practice in wound care and wound healing.

3

In this chapter, you will learn:

1. How the wound environment—the patient—contributes risk factors that may be detrimental not only to the patient's skin (the largest organ of the body), but also to the healing of the wound, particularly a burn wound. As Goethe (1749–1832) wrote, "Nothing in nature is isolated. Nothing is without reference to something else. Nothing achieves meaning apart from that which neighbors it."
2. How the wound care nurse (the clinical expert and educator) works in conjunction with other specialists, staff, and family members to provide and manage personalized wound care plans, educate and empower caretakers, and govern the efficient use of appropriate resources. Without understanding the significance of this component, a facility (or a patient) can end up with "a big problem that demands a big expensive solution," to paraphrase John Kenagy.
3. How to determine whether a wound care product is FDA approved, and how the Centers for Medicare and Medicaid Services (CMS) and the codes of the Healthcare Common Procedure Coding System (HCPCS) process works.

THE PATIENT: THE PHYSIOLOGIC ENVIRONMENT COMPONENT

To understand what fuels a wound, the wound care nurse must understand the wound from the inside out. This knowledge will come from the initial assessment and the patient's history. Take the time to know your patient.

TABLE 1.1 Wound Healing Factors

Risk Factors	Physical Factors	Chemical Factors	Viability Factors
Overall Health:	**Tissue Hydration:**	**Susceptibility Flag for**	**Perfusion Function:**
Comorbidities, such as:	**Osmolality:**	**Wound Infection:**	PaO_2: Normal
Diabetes	Normal	**pH in Blood:**	(90 mmHg on room air)
Steroids	(295 mOsm/kg H_2O)	Neutral (7.4)	Affects wound PO_2
Immunosuppression	Dehydration	**pH on Surface of Skin:**	**Optimizing Perfusion:**
Smoking, obesity	(>295 mOsm/kg H_2O)	Slightly acidic (4.2–5.6)	Cold → Increase warmth.
Mobility:	**Serum Sodium:**	Chemicals in dressings	Fear → Put patient at ease.
Full mobility	Normal	may affect wound pH.	Pain → Medicate.
Limited mobility	(135–150 mEq/L)	A mildly alkaline pH	Discontinue beta blockers.
Immobile	Dehydration	may predispose the	Stop smoking.
Sensory Status:	(>150 mEq/L)	wound to bacterial	Check oxygen status by
Pain	**Serum Albumin:**	infection (Hermans,	transcutaneous oxygen.
Confusion or apathy	(3.5–5.5 g/dL)	1990).	
Unconsciousness or	**Prealbumin:**		
alertness	(15–25 mg/dL)		
	Transferrin:		
	(200–400 mg/dL)		

Continued

TABLE 1.1 Wound Healing Factors *Continued*

Risk Factors	Physical Factors	Chemical Factors	Viability Factors
Nutritional Status: Excellent Adequate Poor or taking nothing by mouth (NPO) **Continence:** Total control Foley or fecal catheter Ostomy or colostomy Incontinent **Causative Factors (6):** Pressure, shear, friction, moisture, neuropathy, circulatory impairment	**Blood Urea Nitrogen:** (7–23 mg/dL) **BUN-to-Creatinine Ratio:** Dehydration (>25:1) Overhydration (<10:1) **Urine Specific Gravity:** (1.035–1.003) Dehydration (>1.010) Overhydration (<1.003) **Body Temperature:** (97.5–99°F) (36.4–37.2°C)	Topical enzymatic debriding agents should not be mixed with silver or heavy metal ions such as mercury—these may inactivate the enzyme.	Check vessel compliance by ankle-brachial index (ABI).

Note: Oxygen status, vessel compliance, and bacterial status are the three physiological parameters that determine the potential for wound healing.

Initial Assessment and History: A Wound Care Nurse Knows the Patient's Baseline

================*FAST FACTS in a NUTSHELL*

Baseline facts help the wound care nurse set realistic, advantageous goals.

- Uncontrolled diabetes can affect wound healing in the areas of nerve damage, lack of physical sensation, poor immune system functioning, higher risk of infections, dry skin, itching, and clogged (hardened) arteries.
- Smoking can affect wound healing by causing inadequate oxygenation. Oxygen is necessary to form collagen, which is necessary to close wounds.
- Pain can affect wound healing by causing vasoconstriction, which slows down the deposition of collagen and protein breakdown, and suppresses the immune system.

Malnutrition

Malnutrition is a nutrition-based disorder in which calories with no nutrients lead to an unbalanced, insufficient, or excessive diet. The three types of malnutrition are:

1. *Marasmus:* Example: people with cancer or chronic obstructive pulmonary disease (COPD), there is gradual weight loss, but serum albumin, pre-albumin, and transferring remain normal.
2. *Kwashiorkor:* Example: poor people in developing countries who have high starch and low protein diets. Onset is rapid, and most commonly, muscle mass is preserved but serum albumin is low, resulting in infections, skin breakdown, edema, and pressure ulcers.
3. *Marasmus-kwashiorkor:* Characterized by morbidity and mortality, with acute onset, most common in hospitalized patients with rapid weight loss and muscle wasting.

TABLE 1.2 The Importance of Nutrition

The Six Major Classes of Nutrients	Role in the Wound Healing Process	Calorie % Needed for Daily Allowance
Carbohydrates	Provide energy and prevent gluconeogenesis.	50–60%
Proteins/Amino Acids	Repair and synthesize enzymes, collagen, and connective tissue. Also aids cell multiplication and production of antibodies.	2025%
Fats/Fatty Acids	Stored triglycerides are concentrated sources and reserves of energy.	20–25%
Vitamins	Vitamin C is essential for collagen synthesis. Vitamin A helps epithelialization, wound closure, and inflammatory response, and counteracts delayed healing in patients on corticosteroids.	60 mg daily 25,000 IU daily for 10 days if on high doses of steroids
Minerals	Copper aids the cross-linking of collagen. Iron aids collagen formation. Magnesium promotes protein synthesis. Zinc aids collagen formation, protein synthesis, blood clotting, and immune system function.	900 mcg daily 8 mg daily 350 mg daily 200–300 mg daily
Water	Aids in hydration and oxygen perfusion. Also acts as a solvent for small molecules such as minerals, vitamins, amino acids, and glucose moving in and out of cell walls.	Patients on air-fluidized beds require an additional 500 mL of fluid daily.

Starvation

Starvation is a condition that develops over a long period of time as a result of a lack of essential nutrients that sustain life. This leads to multiple physiologic and metabolic dysfunctions.

Body Mass Index (BMI)

BMI is a nutritional status tool that uses height and weight to assess whether a person is underweight, has a normal weight, is overweight, or is obese. A BMI between 20 and 25 is normal.

English BMI = [Weight in pounds/(Height in inches)
                        × (Height in inches)] × 703
Metric BMI = [Weight in kilograms/(Height in meters)
                        × (Height in meters)]

Protein Requirements

- New recommendations are between 0.93 and 1.2 g protein/kg/day for adult men.
- Albumin's half life is 12 to 21 days, making it a poor indicator of early malnutrition.
- Pre-albumin has a half life of 2 to 3 days (normal = 15–25 mg/dL).
- Protein is the most important nutrient for a patient who has suffered an injury or trauma.

Dehydration

The minimum daily fluid intake should be 1,500 mL (excluding renal or cardiac stressed patients). Patients with pressure ulcers require at least 30–33 mL/kg/day, with additional fluids to compensate for wound exudates, etc.

Comparing the Needs of Burn Patients

================*FAST FACTS in a NUTSHELL*

- Burn patients require 50–125% increase in food energy.
- Gordon and Goodwin's fluid formula during the first 24–48 hours is:
    mL = 4 × Body weight (kg) × % Body surface area (BSA) of burn
- The Parkland formula for the first 24 hours is:
    Lactated Ringer's solution – 4 mL/kg/% Total body surface area (TBSA)
- The formula for the second 24 hours is one-half the first 24-hour amount
- The amount of fluid resuscitation can be determined from the percentage of BSA involved. "The Rule of 9s" can be used to estimate the percentage of BSA:
    The head = 9%; each arm = 9%; the back and chest = 18% each; each leg = 18%, and the perineum = 1%.

The Harris-Benedict Equation

This equation calculates a person's basal metabolic rate (BMR), which is the amount of energy spent while the body is at complete rest. BMR can otherwise be stated as basal energy expenditure (BEE).

Equation for women:

English BEE = 655 + (4.35 × Weight in pounds)
            + (4.7 × Height in inches) – (4.7 × Age in years)
Metric BEE = 655.1 + (9.563 × Weight in kg)
            + (1.850 × Height in cm) – (4.676 × Age in years)

Equation for men:

English BEE = 66 + (13.7 × Weight in pounds)
            + (5 × Height in inches) – (6.76 × Age in years)

Metric BEE = 66.5 + (13.75 × Weight in kg)
                    + (5.003 × Weight in cm) − (6.775 × Age in years)

Stress Factors

"Stress factors" are used to adjust for burns; they range as follows:

Up to 20% TBS = 1.0–1.5
20–40% TBS = 1.5–1.85
Greater than 40% TBS = 1.85–2.05

Currerí Formula

This is another formula used for the daily caloric requirements of burn patients:

Daily caloric requirements = 25 kcal × Body weight in kg)
                                    + (40 × % TBSA burned)

The maximum TBSA is limited to 50%, but some believe that this formula tends to overestimate caloric needs.

Indirect Calorimetry

Another formula that can be used when a predictive equation is considered too inaccurate (e.g., in the case of limb amputation, or BMI <18 or >30) is:

The respiratory quotient (RQ) = The ratio of CO_2
                                    produced to O_2 consumed

   Results outside of the physiologic range 0.67 to 1.3 reflect a flawed measurement and are to be discarded.

- < 0.7 fat oxidation
- 1.0 glucose use
- 1.0 fat deposition or overfeeding

The clinical value of the measured RQ is limited to that of a marker of test validity and as a measure of tolerance to overfeeding (RQ >1.0) in response to overfeeding.

THE WOUND CARE NURSE COMPONENT

"Unless commitment is made, there are only promises and hopes; but no plans."

—Peter F. Drucker

You will not likely know what patients you will care for each day, or even what wounds they will have. What is your plan? Even more important: What is your goal for your patients today?

The goal of wound care nurses is to raise the bar in wound care management. In light of current health care and economic issues, we need now more than ever to step up and define our position. Wound care teams have the potential to save hospitals money, improve patient outcomes, and raise the "novice-to-expert" bar related to wound care for nurses in every unit with a consultancy team approach. No matter the organization or health care facility, a wound care nurse's responsibilities and roles are threefold:

1. Clinical expert: directing wound management.
2. Educator: empowering staff by teaching them quality wound care.
3. Researcher: improving quality, making evaluations, and collecting data.

Clinical Expert

- Works for and has an understanding of the healthcare system's group purchasing organization (GPO), such as Premier, Novation, HSCA, Consorta, etc.
- Works with the facility's purchasing staff/formulary to balance development of state-of-the-art wound

management formularies and their shared cost-reduction strategy goals.
- Shares responsibility for development and implementation of wound and skin care policies, procedures, and guidelines.

EDUCATOR

- Is able and willing to train students, conduct new employee orientations, and offer novice and staff nurses wound care support.
- Develops a program for organizing wound and skin care products by generic category, and teaches the program and products to the wound care team and staff.
- Understands that wound care can be intimidating, continually changing, and frustrating to staff. The wound care nurse is the resource for problems related to wound and skin care, the sounding board, and the wound care escalation point person.

RESEARCHER

- Understands the scope of "prevalence and incidence" studies, but also appraises quality improvement with statistics such as healing rates, duration times, and percentage of wounds healed.
- Understands and develops (based on the facility) clinical markers for treatment options and treatment guidelines—from aggressive wound care to palliative care.
- Observes the wound care team and develops care maps to elevate novice team members to consultancy experts who can empower others.

==*FAST FACTS in a NUTSHELL*

Two organizations established for credentialing specialized wound management:

- The American Academy of Wound Management: www.aawm.org
- The Wound, Ostomy, and Continence Nurses Association: www.wocn.org

THE DRESSING MANUFACTURE COMPONENT

"A product takes a long, expensive, and rigorous journey to go from a manufacturer's think tank to the hands of the end-user. Vague ideas and concepts are molded and moved into the research and development pipeline where, over time, a product is perfected. Once the product has been refined and tested, it is strategically marketed so that it will find its way to the targeted end-user."

—Gwen Turnbull

Along with vague ideas and concepts that begin the process of perfecting a product, new or old terms—description labels— are continuously being created or resurfacing. For instance, *evidence-based medicine* (EBM) is a term that has resurfaced, and it should not be taken for granted.

==*FAST FACTS in a NUTSHELL*

Question: How do you know that a wound-care product that you are using is what it claims to be?

Answer: The U.S. FDA establishes and monitors the quality as well as violations of dressing manufactures, detailed on 510(k) forms. It is up to the wound care nurse to find out if a product is FDA approved.

Continued

Continued

Question: Who pays your facility for services and treatments rendered? Do you understand how the CMS fit into this picture?

Answer: The CMS pays health care facilities for wound care products, services, and technologies based on codes of the Healthcare Common Procedure Coding System (HCPCS).

Following is a brief example of how the CMS and the HCPCS process works. The CMS partnered with the Agency for Healthcare Research and Quality (AHRQ) to commission a review of negative pressure wound therapy (NPWT) devices. The purpose of the review was to provide information to the CMS for consideration of an HCPCS code, meaning that the CMS would pay for the devices based on this code. Section 154(c)(3) of the Medicare Improvements for Patient and Providers Act of 2008 (MIPPA) called for the Secretary of Health and Human Services to perform an evaluation of the HCPCS codes for the NPWT devices. After this process was finalized, a code was issued.

This process can be quite complicated. As Laurence J. Peter said, "Some problems are so complex that you have to be highly intelligent and well informed just to be undecided about them." The minimum information that you will want to have on hand regarding each of your formulary products are: an HCPCS code, an MSDS sheet, a product insert (a user guide from the manufacturer that includes a description, directions for use and removal of the dressing, indications, and instructions for frequency of change), and relevant studies.

I wish I could say that I have never known of any money-making scams related to wound care products; sadly, I have. How does one tell whether a product is legitimate? Reputable wound care products are FDA approved, and the manufacturers will provide proof of this. Knowing and understanding your products are another way of being your patients' advocate.

═══════════════════════ *FAST FACTS in a NUTSHELL*

**Establish a Wound and Skin Care
Product Formulary notebook.**

Supplies Needed: A notebook with plastic sleeves and alphabet dividers.

• For each product, Alphabetically place the product insert, MSDS sheet, the product insert, and studies in a sleeve.

This is a good Scavenger Hunt game for new wound care team members to play, as each member should have his or her own such notebook as a learning and teaching tool.

2

Understanding Wound Etiology

INTRODUCTION

This chapter is about becoming proficient in understanding wound pathophysiology, identifying the cause of a wound, understanding the normal wound healing process, and knowing the factors that influence this process. The ultimate goal for the wound care nurse is to optimize the healing process, maximize functional performance, and improve the quality of life for the patient whenever possible.

In this chapter, you will learn:

1. The characteristics of acute and chronic wounds and their significant differences.
2. The three phases of wound healing and the three types of scar tissue.
3. The body's defenses against infection and signs that tissue has been invaded to the point of infection.
4. What a bioburden is and how it affects wounds and wound healing.
5. How to diagnose wound infections and manage wound odors.

THE DIFFERENCES BETWEEN CHRONIC AND ACUTE WOUNDS

Description of Chronic Wounds

- Chronic wounds usually result from recurring pathologic tissue damage.
- Examples of chronic wounds include:
  - Pressure ulcers
  - Diabetic ulcers
  - Vascular ulcers
- These wounds are categorized as full-thickness wounds.
- Chronic wound healing (or closure) occurs differently from acute wound healing. The recurring tissue damage "fools" the wound healing process by "crying wolf" to the wound healing cascade and skips the process of hemostasis (vasoconstriction, blood clotting, and fibrinolysis).
- These wounds proceed directly to the three phases of chronic wound healing (inflammation, proliferative, and remodeling).

Description of Acute Wounds

- Acute wounds begin with an injury to the skin that causes bleeding, triggers clot formation, and results in the wound healing cascade.
- Examples of acute wounds include:
  - Surgical wounds closed with glue, sutures, staples, or tape
  - Trauma wounds (such as road rash)
  - Burn wounds
- Acute wounds with no complications or infections heal by primary intention. This means that the epidermal and dermal layers (epithelial, endothelial, and connective tissue) reproduce in a process called regeneration.
- Acute wound closure usually occurs within 72 hours.
- Surgical wound closure occurs as the reproduced epithelial cells migrate, in a leapfrog fashion, from the wound edges inward.

- Burn and trauma wound closure occurs as the epithelial cells migrate from sebaceous glands, sweat glands, and hair follicles.

THE THREE PHASES OF CHRONIC WOUND HEALING

Inflammatory Phase

- This phase is characterized by the cleaning of the wound, which averages 2 to 5 days.
- It involves inflammatory cells: neutrophils, macrophages, and lymphocytes.
- All three types of inflammatory cells destroy bacteria via vasodilation and a process called phagocytosis.
- Macrophages come from monocytes, and they provide cytokines and growth factors.
- Common terms associated with chronic wound healing include matrix metalloproteases (MMPs) and tissue inhibitors of metalloproteases (TIMPs), especially elevated matrix metalloproteases (MMPs) (protease levels) and deficient (TIMPs) (protease inhibitor levels).
- Expected symptoms include discomfort, ¼ inch of redness around the wound edges, and swelling.

Proliferation Phase

- This phase is characterized by tissue granulation. Typically, one can tell that a wound is in the proliferative phase when 50% or more of the wound is granulated and contracting inward.
- The proliferation phase involves the production of granulation tissue, wound contraction, and epithelialization, which can last for a period of 2 days to 3 weeks.
- It involves proteoglycans (PGs), fibroblasts, collagen, and glycosaminoglycans (GAGs) that fill the wound

bed and produce new capillaries through the process of angiogenesis.
- Contraction occurs as the wound starts to heal and the tissue and skin pull together.
- Finally, the wound is resurfaced by epithelial cells, which completes the last component of this phase, known as epithelialization.

Remodeling Phase

This phase is characterized by the formation of new collagen, which is required for building tensile strength and, eventually, scar formation; the time period can range from 3 weeks to 2 years.

The collagen deposition and remodeling cause the new skin (scar tissue) to reach a tensile strength of approximately 80%.

$=$ *FAST FACTS in a NUTSHELL*

How to tell the differences between granulation tissue and epithelium.

- Healthy granulation tissue is bright beefy red, shiny, and bumpy. It bleeds easily.
- New epithelium changes from a shiny, granulation look to a polished pink sheen as blood vessels heal and are not needed in the formation of scar tissue.
- The production of granulation tissue is similar to the process of wet concrete setting in a form and losing its sheen as it dries, with epithelium being like the top flat layer that is "floated" smooth.
- A wound may look as if it has healed, but may require time for the collagen deposition to reach the tensile strength of scar tissue that is required to resist breakdown, similar to model airplane pieces that have been glued and need time to set.

TYPES OF WOUND CLOSURE

Primary Intention

These are wounds that are approximated with sutures, staples, glue, or tape. Examples include surgical wounds and lacerations.

Secondary Intention

These wounds heal by granulation and contraction. An example is a chronic wound, such as a pressure ulcer.

Tertiary (Delayed Primary) Intention

These are wounds that are purposely kept open for observation of possible contamination, draining, cleaning, and debridement if necessary. Typically, tertiary intention wounds are surgical wounds. Usually within 3 to 7 days the patient returns to surgery for closure of the wound. An example is a dehisced or eviscerated abdominal wound.

TYPES OF SCAR TISSUE

Hypertrophic Scars

These scars extend above surrounding skin. They are smaller than keloid scars and usually fade with time.

Keloid Scars

These scars extend not only above but also beyond wounds, burns, or incisions. Keloids are considered benign tumors (never malignant). People who have darkly pigmented skin are more prone to develop keloid scar tissue than are people with lighter skin pigmentation. It is estimated that keloid scarring occurs in about 10% of men and women.

- *Treatment Options:* Surgery usually stimulates more scar tissue, making more keloids. Often, better options such as foam dressings, silicone gel pads, compression garments, or cortisone shots, may be successful in reducing keloid scars.

Contractures

Contractures are proliferations of scar tissue and normal tissue that draw up and pull into wounds associated with burns. Contractures affect joint mobility, sometimes to the extent of severely reducing joint flexibility

- *Treatment Options:* Splints, range of motion exercises, specific positioning, and/or compression garments.

Note: Contractures are not to be confused with the contraction process in wound healing.

═══════════════════════════*FAST FACTS in a NUTSHELL*

Physiology of Fetal Wound Healing

- It is a known fact that fetal skin can heal without scar formation, but there is still much to learn about the process, which is related to biomedical ethics.
- A fascinating factor that may contribute to the non-scarring of fetal skin is the amniotic fluid, which is rich in hyaluronic acid (HA), fibronectin, and growth factors.
- HA is a key component of the extracellular matrix (ECM) and promotes cell proliferation, tissue regeneration, and repair.

INFECTIONS AND BIOBURDENS

An infection occurs when microorganisms (pathogens) colonize to the point of invading the host tissue. Pathogens can originate through contact with chemicals, bacteria, viruses, and contaminated water. Skin in a healthy state protects the body from the invasion of pathogens through its stratum corneum layer. Additional body defenses against the invasion of pathogens include secretions from the sebaceous glands and the immune system. Some pathogens are part of the body's natural flora and become harmful only after invading the tissue. These are opportunistic pathogens, so named because they attack the body's defenses when an opportunity presents itself, such as during surgery, in the event of trauma to the skin/body, or through an existing wound.

Contamination is the presence of pathogens on the surface of the skin or a wound. *Colonization* occurs when contaminants multiply significantly and the body's immune system is overwhelmed. Signs of inflammation become apparent: redness, heat, and/or drainage.

Bioburdens

A bioburden is the number of contaminating microbes, (organisms, germs, pathogens) on the surface of a wound.

Biofilms

A biofilm is the ECM structure that attaches itself to a wound's surface tissue (necrotic or living) and protects microbes from the host's defenses, similar to how an egg yolk is within the egg white and is protected by it. A biofilm structure attaches itself very firmly to the surrounding environmental surface of the wound. The biofilm must be scrubbed off the wound; simply spritzing wound cleanser or pouring sterile water on the wound is not effective.

Several factors lead from wound contamination to community (biofilm) colonization to infection. These include:

- Pathogens that are resistant to traditional antibiotic therapy
- The type of pathogen species present
- The variety of different species present
- The interaction of different species with each other
- The capability of the host's immune response system
- The presence of a biofilm community

Treatment of Biofilms

Recent research has identified some treatments that effectively target biofilms.

- *Cadexomer Iodine:* destroys biofilm structures and kills *Staphylococcus aureus* within biofilms.
- *Silver:* very effective against mature biofilms of *Pseudomonas aeruginosa.*
- *Honey: a* bactericidal for all strains of bacteria.
- *Maggots:* treat and prevent biofilms from forming. It is important to take into account how this treatment choice might affect the patient.

═══════════════════════*FAST FACTS in a NUTSHELL*

Wound Agents

Bactericidal: An agent that destroys bacteria.
Bacteriostatic: An agent that is able to prevent new bacteria from growing or multiplying but does not destroy bacteria that are already present.

Deep Sternal Wound Infections

Surgical-site infections are the most common nosocomial (hospital-acquired) infections among surgical patients. The national incidence of deep sternal wound infections ranges from 0.5% to 5% and is associated with a morbidity and mortality rate of 14%. The Centers for Disease Control and Prevention (CDC) define a deep sternal wound infection as an infection involving incisional deep soft tissue occurring within 30 days of an operation.

═══════════════════════════*FAST FACTS in a NUTSHELL*

Clinical Indications for a Wound Culture

- Systemic signs of infection, fever, or leukocytosis
- Sudden high glucose
- Pain in the neuropathic extremity
- Lack of healing of a clean-looking wound after 2 weeks

Signs and Symptoms of Infection at the Wound Site

- Pain or tenderness
- Excess drainage
- Change in color
- Redness
- Warmth around the wound
- Unusual odor
- Swelling or firmness

Diagnostic Follow-up for Confirming Wound Infection

There are several methods of diagnosing an infection. Quantitative tissue biopsies, needle aspiration, and superficial swab samples are the most common lab tests for diagnosing an infection. The results believed to confirm an infection range between 10 to 100,000 pathogen cells per gram of wound tissue (depending upon how virulent the organisms are). All chronic wounds are contaminated; therefore, newer research suggests diagnosing wound infection based on clinical signs and establishing a host-manageable bioburden. Nevertheless, it is important that specimens be taken from healthy-looking tissue.

Tissue Biopsies

A tissue biopsy is considered the most reliable method of diagnosing a wound infection. However, tissue biopsies are invasive and expensive. A tissue biopsy is not cost effective when signs/symptoms of an infection are apparent.

Needle Aspiration

In needle aspiration, fluid is obtained from multiple insertions using a 22-gauge needle and a 10-cc syringe. Needle aspiration is thought to be the best technique for tissue-fluid or abscess-related wounds. One would expect the number of organisms from needle aspiration to be less than the number in a culture on a tissue biopsy.

Swab Cultures

A swab culture is taken by swabbing the surface of a wound. Although it is the most commonly used method of diagnosing a wound infection, swabbing techniques are unreliable because a swab is easily contaminated during the culture collecting process.

- The Levine technique is believed to be most reflective of tissue bioburden. Obtaining this type of swab culture consists of rotating a swab over a 1 cm² area with sufficient pressure to express fluid from within the wound tissue.

════════════════════════════════*FAST FACTS in a NUTSHELL*

It is important to know that it is possible for wound-culture reports to have false results. The variety of false results include:

- **False-Positive:** Organisms are present on the surface that was cultured but are not present in the tissue.
- **False-Negative:** Organisms are not present on the surface that was cultured but are present in the tissue.
- **Chance-Agreement:** The surface area and tissue have same result (the probability is not likely).

The germ is nothing. It is the terrain in which it is found that is everything.

—Louis Pasteur

WOUND ODORS

Professional Behavior for Managing Wound Odors

Many wounds are accompanied by odors, which may be quite unpleasant. To avoid embarrassing patients in such instances, it is important to be prepared to manage wound odors in a professional, compassionate, and empathetic manner. Take precautions to address the potential for your experiencing an involuntary gag response or some other equally embarrassing reaction. Some strategies to employ might include:

- Wearing a mask when performing wound care
- Using a scent inside the mask such as that emitted by chewing gum, peppermints, or perfume to help prevent involuntary gagging
- Avoiding behaviors that communicate disrespect; for example, not commenting on wound odors and

refraining from wrinkling the nose or making other unpleasant expressions.
- Remember, your patient is suffering already, and part of that suffering may result from the patient's perception of how you (the caretaker) react to his or her odor.

Identify and Understand Odor Sources

- Wounds with bioburden (e.g., *Clostridium, Proteus, Klebeilla, Pseudomonas*, and bacteria)
- Wounds with necrotic tissue, slough/pus (e.g., pressure ulcers, vascular ulcers, and diabetic ulcers)
- Drain sites
- Fistulas
- Ostomies (e.g., colostomies, ileostomies, and urostomies)
- End-stage wounds (e.g., fungating wounds)
- Certain types of dressings or inappropriate dressings (e.g., hydrocolloids)
- Poor hygiene

Recommendations for Effective Wound Odor Control

- When using gauze dressings, notify the physician regarding a heavily draining wound, and request an order to clean the wound and change the dressing more often, as needed. Gauze dressings do not control odor.
- Change linens and patient gowns daily and more often, if needed.
- Bathe the patient more often, if needed.
- Take soiled linens and dressings completely out of and away from the patient's room.
- Use a deodorant for the patient and a room spray that eliminates odors (and not just masks them).
- Use the correct size and type of ostomy bag, deodorant, and skin sealant.

- Address the cause of the odor (remove/debride wound-bed contaminants and control infection).
- Consider a different Dressing.

Recommendations for Effective End-Stage Draining Wound Odor Control

- Use charcoal dressings, antimicrobial dressings, and silver sulfadiazine (SSD) dressings.
- Use cat litter under the patient's bed, scented candles, a coffee filter with dry coffee in it, and aromatherapy.
- After dressing the wound, put baking soda **on top** of the dressing—not on the wound.
- Finely crush metronidazole (Flagyl) or open 375 mg capsules and sprinkle this antibiotic in the wound.

3

Assessing and Documenting Wounds

INTRODUCTION

All assessment is perpetual work in progress.

—Linda Suske

Do not allow making assessments to intimidate you. Think about making assessments in terms of the analogy that just because you've seen one human face doesn't mean that you've seen them all, or that you will ever see them all. However, as Vince Lombardi said, "Practice does not make perfect. Only perfect practice makes perfect." Continually making assessments will improve your skills and make you more effective in developing your treatment plans. Take time with your assessments, and really scrutinize what you are assessing.

In this chapter, you will learn:

1. How to assess various aspects of pain by asking the patient questions about his or her pain and by using a pain scale.
2. How to manage the patient's pain by eliminating it or providing analgesia.

3. How to obtain a full history of the patient, as this will be the first indicator of his or her intrinsic ability to heal.
4. How to document the features of a wound, its edges, and the surrounding skin to make and meet an early goal for the patient's expected wound care outcome, and how to document the anatomical location of the wound, relevant dates, and related information on a wound assessment form.

RECOGNIZING AND MANAGING PAIN

An accurate wound assessment is the first step in a wound care plan. The assessment provides baseline data and records ongoing changes—which measure the effectiveness of the treatment plan—and interventions related to the progression of the wound's status. The mnemonic KISS, which means, "Keep it simple, silly" is a good guideline for wound assessment. Another mnemonic to help you make sure that all the elements are covered as quickly as possible is PRIORITY.

═══════════════════════════*FAST FACTS in a NUTSHELL*

The P R I O R I T Y Wound Assessment Mnemonic

- P = Patient's pain
- R = Recognize underlying conditions
- I = Initial inspection
- O = Other locations
- R = Record wound characteristics
- I = Infection
- T = Treatment goals
- Y = You observe the wound

Pain is inevitable. Suffering is optional.

—Anonymous

If you were to excel in only one type of assessment, it should be accurate and continuous pain assessment. It is our responsibility as clinicians to identify and treat pain. As Margo McCaffery, MS, RN-BC, FAAN, said, "A patient's pain is what they say it is"—plain and simple—and should never be neglected. The American Pain Society identifies pain as "the fifth vital sign."

Basics of Pain Assessment

Asking the patient the following questions will help you to assess his or her pain: Where is the pain? Does it radiate? Obtain further information from the patient about his or her pain:

- *Rate the Pain*: Have the patient rate his or her pain using a pain scale.
- *Facial Expression*: An absence of expression or response does not mean that the patient is free of pain.
- *Time*: When did the pain start, and is it ongoing?
- *Kind of Pain*: Is it aching, burning, cramping, deep, sensitive, and so on?
- *Cause of Pain*: Is it edema, dressing changes, debridement, infection, position changes, etc.?

Pain Scales

- *Visual Analog Scale (VAS)*: This is a 10-cm long line with the words *no pain* at one end and *worst possible pain* at the other end.

The Visual Analog Scale (VAS)

0|_____|10

No Pain   Worst Possible Pain

Source: D'Arcy, Y. (2011). *Compact clinical guide to chronic pain management.* New York: Springer Publishing.

- *FACES Pain Rating Scale*: Preferred for use with children.

Wong-Baker FACES Pain Rating Scale

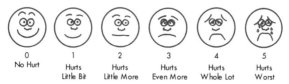

Brief word instructions: Point to each face using the words to describe the pain intensity. Ask the child to choose face that best describes own pain and record the appropriate number.

Original instructions: Explain to the person that each face is for a person who feels happy because he has no pain (hurt) or sad because he has some or a lot of pain. Face 0 is very happy because he doesn't hurt at all. Face 1 hurts just a little bit. Face 2 hurts a little more. Face 3 hurts even more. Face 4 hurts a whole lot. Face 5 hurts as much as you can imagine, although you don't have to be crying to feel this bad. Ask the person to choose the face that best desribes how he is feeling.

Rating scale is recommended for persons age 3 years and older.

Source: From Hockenberry MJ, Wilson D: *Wong's essentials of pediatric nursing,* ed. 8, St. Louis, 2009, Mosby. Used with permission. Copyright Mosby.

- *Numeric Rating Scale (NRS)*: Commonly considered the gold standard, this is an 11-point Likert-type scale where zero means *no pain* and 10 means *worst possible pain.*

Numeric Rating Scale (NRS)

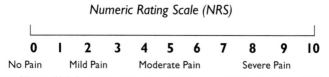

Source: D'Arcy, Y. (2011). Compact clinical guide to chronic pain management. New York: Springer Publishing.

Pain Management: Be Confident With Providing Analgesia

The goal of pain management is to identify the cause of pain, eliminate the cause, and/or provide analgesia. The World Health Organization (WHO) developed a three-step analgesic ladder, proceeding from nonopioids (with or without adjuvants) up to the opioids (with or without adjuvants) as needed to achieve an adequate and acceptable level of pain

TABLE 3.1	The WHO Pain Relief Ladder	
Patient Report of Pain Level	**Class of Pain Medication to Use**	**Use of Adjuvant Medication**
Step One: 1–3 (mild pain)	Nonopioid Examples: aspirin, nonsteroidal anti-inflammatory drugs (NSAIDs)	With or without an adjuvant
Step Two: 4–6 (moderate pain)	Weak opioid Examples: codeine, propoxyphene	With or without an adjuvant
Step Three: 7–10 (severe pain)	Strong opioid Examples: morphine, fentanyl patch	With or without an adjuvant

relief to the patient. The WHO pain ladder is a good guideline for mild-to-severe pain. The WHO pain ladder's key principles are "by mouth," "by the clock," "by the ladder," "for the individual," and "attention to detail."

Adjuvants treat side effects and provide additional analgesia. Examples include antidiarrheal agents, antidepressants, antipsychotics, laxatives, antiemetics, anticonvulsants, and corticosteroids. The clinician should reevaluate adjuvants every time analgesics are changed.

The WHO guidelines state that, "Relief of psychological, social and spiritual problems is paramount. Attempting to relieve pain without addressing the patient's non-physical concerns is likely to lead to frustration and failure."

OBTAINING A PATIENT'S HISTORY

An expert wound care nurse does not just simply slap a dressing on a wound. Instead, the wound care nurse defines the patient's expected wound care outcome. The goal should be realistic and established early. The patient's history is the first indicator of his or her intrinsic ability to heal.

There are three parts of a patient's wound care history:

1. The patient's health (nutritional, psychological, and cultural history; causative factors; and risk factors, such as disease processes, compliancy, care setting, economic status, medications, home life or homelessness, occupation, and smoking and/or any other addictions).
2. The physical assessment (systems review).
3. The wound history.

=========================*FAST FACTS in a NUTSHELL*

Questions to ask in obtaining a wound history:

- When did you first notice the wound? Is this the first time you've had it?
- Does it hurt? Where? How? (Use a pain scale.)
- Has it changed in size, odor, and/or appearance?
- Who takes care of it? You or a caretaker?
- What have you been putting on the wound?

There are two easy tests to be done during an initial assessment: one for arterial perfusion of the lower legs, and the other for protective sensation of the feet.

1. *Ankle-Brachial Index (ABI)*: A simple comparison of perfusion pressures in the lower legs with those in the upper arms.
2. *Semmes–Weinstein Monofilament Examination*: A simple test of protective sensation of the feet. The Semmes-Weinstein Microfilament test is used to assess the degree of sensation on the plantar surface of feet (see figure 7.4 on page 103)

Name_____
Patient FIN#_____
Date of Birth_____
Age_____
M/F
Room #_____
Consult Type_____
Date of Assessment_____
Assessed by_____

WOUND ASSESSMENT FORM
Referring physician_____ Diagnosis
Medication allergies_____
Skin/wound product sensitivities_____
Date wound occurred_____ Date admitted_____
Cause of wound _____

Acute Traumatic: Open/Closed	**Acute Surgical:** Open/Closed	**Chronic: Present Over 6 WK?** (Y/N)
☐ Abrasion	☐ Surgical	☐ Fungating wound
☐ Laceration	☐ Dehiscence	
☐ Crush	☐ Graft	☐ Ulcer
☐ Skin tear category	☐ Donor site	☐ Pressure ulcer
☐ 1 ☐ 2 ☐ 3	☐ Debridement	stage ☐ I ☐ II
☐ Hematoma present		☐ III ☐ IV
☐ Burn: –Type		

_____

FIGURE 3.1   Sample Wound Assessment Form

Continued

Continued

Assessment	Treatment
Patient's perception of wound pain (circle one) Pre-dressing (min.) 1 2 3 4 5 6 7 8 9 10 (max.) Post-dressing (min.) 1 2 3 4 5 6 7 8 9 10 (max.)	**Medicated prior to dressing change?** ☐ Yes ☐ No
Exudate amount: ☐ Dry ☐ Primary dressing is unmarked ☐ Moist ☐ Primary dressing is lightly marked ☐ Soaking ☐ Primary dressing is saturated	**Treatment goal:** ☐ Control pain ☐ Debridement ☐ Control exudate ☐ Encourage granulation ☐ Rehydration ☐ Protection ☐ Reduce bacterial burden ☐ Palliative wound care
Exudate color: ☐ Clear/amber (normal) ☐ Green (infection) ☐ Pink or red (blood stained) ☐ Cloudy/milky/creamy (purulent) ☐ Yellow or brown (slough) ☐ Gray (silver dressing) ☐ Other_____ _____☐ N/A	Dressing schedule: ☐ Daily ☐ 2× day ☐ 3× day ☐ Weekly ☐ 2× week (M T W T F) ☐ 3× week (M T W T F S) ☐ Other
Exudate consistency: ☐ Thick ☐ Sticky ☐ Thin ☐ Runny ☐ Serous (normal) ☐ Other ☐ /A	**Cleansing method:** ☐ saline ☐ sterile water ☐ Wound cleanser ☐ Swab ☐ Irrigation ☐ Shower ☐ Other_____

Continued

Wound edge:
☐ Advancing ☐ Tracking/ undermining ☐ Rolled/raised ☐ Macerated ☐ Fragile/red ☐ Firm/ epithelializing

Surrounding skin temperature:
☐ Normal ☐ Warm ☐ Cool ☐ Hot

Surrounding skin appearance:
☐ Healthy/intact ☐ Thin/fragile ☐ Macerated ☐ Excoriated ☐ Venous staining ☐ Bruising ☐ Eczema ☐ Cellulitis

Wound bed:
☐ Epithelializing (pink)
☐ Granulating (red)
☐ Slough (yellow)
☐ Necrotic/eschar (black)
☐ Hypergranulation
☐ Other_____

Wound measurements: (record length head to toe)
Width_____ cm
Length_____ cm
Depth_____ cm
Undermining_____ cm

Care to surrounding skin:
☐ Skin preps ☐ Skin protectant ☐ Barrier cream
☐ Other_____

Primary dressing:
☐ Calcium alginate
☐ Foam
☐ Hydrogel
☐ Hydrocolloid
☐ Transparent film
☐ Cadexomer iodine
☐ Charcoal
☐ Antimicrobial dressing
☐ NPWT ☐ Other
_____

Secondary dressing:
☐ Foam ☐ Gauze
☐ Transparent Film
☐ Non-adherent dressing ☐ Hydrocolloid
☐ Other _____
_____
_____

Wound photographed?
Yes ☐ No ☐

FIGURE 3.1   Sample Wound Assessment Form

Continued

Continued

Wound Location

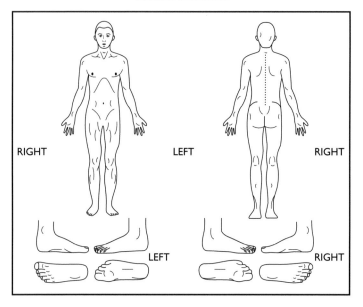

FIGURE 3.1   Sample Wound Assessment Form

DOCUMENTING A WOUND

A wound care nurse must document the key features of a wound, the wound edges, and the surrounding skin as part of the plan to make and meet an early goal for the patient's expected wound care outcome. In addition to this information, other relevant information should be documented on a wound assessment form.

Surrounding Skin: Assess the surrounding skin for color, temperature, and general skin condition.

• Is the surrounding skin intact, erythematous, edematous, marked by induration, warm, cool, and/or dry?
• Is the surrounding skin normal, warm, cool, or hot?

- Is the surrounding skin thin fragile, macerated, or excoriated?
- Are there signs of venous staining, bruising, or cellulitis?

Wound Edges: Assess the age and type of wound.

- *Acute Traumatic*: Assess whether the wound is open or closed; an abrasion, laceration, or crush injury; a skin tear (category 1, 2, or 3); or a burn.
- *Acute Surgical*: Assess whether the edges are attached or not, whether the incision is approximated or open, and whether sutures or staples are intact or calloused.
- *Chronic (Present for More Than 6 Weeks)*: Assess whether it is a fungating ulcer or pressure ulcer (Stage I, II, III, or IV).
- *Maceration*: Assess for the presence of macerated skin, which appears shriveled, like hands that have been in a swimming pool or bath water for a long time. Don't confuse maceration with slough. Maceration does not come off; slough does.
- *Epibole*: The edges of healed skin (epidermis) have rolled under to the point that epithelial cells cannot migrate from the wound edges. This requires removal of the edges, which may be achieved by scrubbing the edges until they bleed and applying silver nitrate to the edges, or by surgical excision.
- *Sinus Tracts*: Observe for sinus tracts, which are infection drainage pathways from deep tissue and/or bone to an opening on the surface.
- *Tunneling*: Assess for tunneling, which is a passageway underneath the skin that can extend in any direction through soft tissue and results in dead space and the threat of abscess formation.
- *Undermining*: Evaluate the wound edges for signs of undermining, which is tissue destruction that extends under and along the wound edges.
- *Fistula*: Observe for a fistula, which is an abnormal connection between an organ, vessel, or intestine and another structure.

FAST FACTS in a NUTSHELL

Terminology for Documenting the Anatomic Locations of Wounds For Hands
Palmar: toward the palm
Dorsal: opposite of plantar
For Limbs
Proximal: toward the center/nearest
Distal: away from the center
For Feet
Plantar: toward the bottom
Dorsal: opposite of palmar

For Body
Medial: toward the middle
Dorsal: located near
Posterior: the back/underside
Superior: the top/up
Anterior: the front/top
Inferior: below/down
Lateral: toward the side
For Trochanter, Ischium, Sacrum, and Coccyx
Think of the pelvic girdle's shape as a butterfly.
The sacrum is the upper butterfly body part (pressure point when lying on one's back).
The coccyx is the lower butterfly body part (pressure point when sitting in a chair).
The trochanters are the upper tips of the wings (pressure point when lying on one's side).
The ischial tuberosities are the lower tips of the wings (pressure points when one is sitting).

Wound Bed Tissue: Examine the wound bed tissue itself for the presence of granulation, epithelialization, slough, necrosis, or hypergranulation.

- *Granulation*: Tissue appears red: Is it present? If so, in what amount?

- *Epithelialization*: This is regenerated epidermis on the wound bed surface; it can appear moist, dry, and pink.
- *Necrosis*: Tissue can be slough (yellow) or eschar (black). Assess the percentage
- *Hypergranulation*: This is an excess of granulation tissue believed to be stimulated from myofibroblasts or exposure of a dressing that is too moist.
- *Sepsis*: Assess for the potential of local or systemic infection. Indicators of local infection include odor. Document the nature of the odor: strong, foul, pungent, fecal, musty, or sweet?

Exudate: Evaluate the nature and amount of exudate:

- Is it serosanguineous, sanguineous, serous (normal), or purulent?
- Is there none, or is it moderate or heavy?
- Observe the dressing. Is it dry (unmarked), moist (lightly marked), or soaking (saturated)?
- Assess the color of exudates: Is it clear/amber (normal); pink/red (blood stained); yellow/brown (slough); green (infection); cloudy/milky/creamy (purulent); or gray (silver dressing).

Shape: Identify the shape of the wound: Is it oval, round, or irregular?

Size: Assess and document the size of the wound by measuring its length × width × depth; this provides a consistent basis for ongoing evaluation to determine the effectiveness of treatment and the rate of healing.

- *Width and Length Measurement*: Measure the width and length of the wound in centimeters (cm), not inches. Measure the greatest width and length of the wound, perpendicular to each other, using the clock method, associating the head of the patient with 12:00 on a clock. Other methods to employ include tracing and photographing.

- *Depth Measurement*: Determine the depth of the wound using a cotton swab (preferably premarked with measurements). Hold it in place in the deepest area of the wound, lay another cotton swab across the top of the wound, and gently roll this swab until it makes contact with the inserted swab. Pick up the inserted swab with your fingertips; where the two swabs met is the measurement used for depth.

DOCUMENTATION OF ASSESSMENT FINDINGS

It is important to document all of your assessment findings in the patient's health record, using a wound assessment form if possible (Figure 3.1).

Complete documentation includes the following information:

- The initial assessment date and improvement/ deteriorating/healed dates.
- Notifications to physicians with dates.
- Supportive therapy (compression, off-loading, mattress/ bed for pressure relief).
- Referrals.
- The patient's perceptions/reactions.

4

Debriding Wounds

INTRODUCTION

Wound debridement is effective in reducing the bioburden of a wound, in controlling and/or preventing a wound infection, and in removing necrotic tissue, such as eschar or slough. There are several types of wound debridement, one or more of which may be used to access healthy tissue underneath the wound and to interrupt the viscous chronic wound cycle. Debridement choices can range from sharp, autolytic, enzymatic, chemical, and mechanical debridement to biodebridement (use of maggots). Wound care nurses must become familiar with the advantages and disadvantages of these debridement approaches.

In this chapter, you will learn:

1. Indications for debridement and how it facilitates wound healing.
2. The types of gangrene and the importance of not removing dry gangrene (stable eschar).
3. The methods of debridement, how they are classified, and their actual mechanism of action.
4. How to choose the most suitable debridement method based on advantages and disadvantages.
5. Why wet-to-dry is not the current "gold standard"—with important pros and cons to consider.

INDICATIONS FOR DEBRIDEMENT

Debridement is indicated for any chronic or acute wound with necrotic tissue such as eschar or slough. Debridement is also indicated if foreign bodies or signs and symptoms of infection are present, such as edema, erythema, fluctuance, and/or discharge. No wound that contains necrotic tissue will heal. Wounds that are *not* candidates for debridement include decubiti wounds with dry, stable, black eschar and wounds resulting from peripheral arterial disease (PAD) or autoimmune conditions.

═══════════════════════════════════════*FAST FACTS in a NUTSHELL*

Contraindications for Debridement

Debridement is not indicated for:

1. Clean wounds.
2. Dry, stable, black eschar on pressure ulcers that cover the healed skin and show no signs or symptoms of infection (Agency for Health Care Policy and Research, 1994).
3. Dry, stable, ischemic wounds resulting from PAD, autoimmune conditions, or *Pyoderma gangrenosum*.

Gangrene

Gangrene is the death of tissue resulting from an obstruction in the blood supply to the tissue. It can occur in skin, muscles, or organs (most commonly in the arms and legs).

There are three types of gangrene:

1. *Dry Gangrene*: This is known as stable eschar and is caused by a progressive reduction of blood flow through the arteries.
   • It progresses slowly.
   • It usually is not infected.
2. *Wet Gangrene*: An untreated bacterial infection causes a sudden stop in arterial blood flow.
   • It allows the multiplication and invasion of the bacteria into muscle tissue.

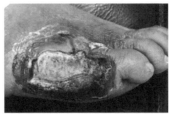

Wet Gangrene

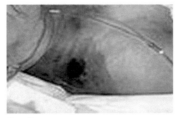

Gas Gangrene

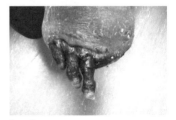

Dry Gangrene

FIGURE 4.1 Gangrene Photos

3. *Gas Gangrene*: This is a type of wet gangrene caused by the bacteria known as *Clostridium*.
   - *Clostridium* grows in the absence of oxygen and produces poisonous toxins and gas.
   - It is most common in wounds contaminated with dirt.

Signs and Symptoms of Gangrene

It is important to assess and treat wet and gas gangrene quickly because the infection spreads rapidly. The patch of damaged skin turns pale, then red (or bronze), and finally purple (or dark red). The skin quickly becomes warm, edematous, and extremely painful. The evolving wound will have a brownish-red or bloody discharge and a foul-smelling odor. The damaged tissue is completely destroyed. Once it is destroyed, the tissue must be removed immediately.

Treatment for Gangrene

The treatment goal for dry gangrene is to keep the tissue dry. Intervention strategies include:

- Protect stable necrotic heels of the feet by leaving them open to air or wrapping them in dry gauze.
- For off-load heels, the dry eschar acts as a natural barrier to infection.
- Check between the toes often and keep them clean; apply alcohol pads between the toes to keep them dry.
- Monitor frequently for signs of change.
- The treatment goal is to prevent trauma and avoid infection.

Effective management of wet and gas gangrene is to treat the underlying cause:

- Use antibiotics for surrounding tissue.
- Hyperbaric oxygen therapy may be a good option.
- The last resort is amputation of the affected body part.

TYPES OF DEBRIDEMENT

The Four Kinds of Sharp Debridement

1. *Conservative Sharp (or Selective) Debridement*: This is the most aggressive type of debridement that wound care nurses can perform. Also called selective debridement, conservative sharp debridement is considered within a nurse's scope of practice in most states, as the procedure (done correctly) is not aggressive enough to risk the patient's viable tissue. The wound care nurse uses sterile forceps ("pick-ups"), scissors, and a scalpel to remove loosely adherent, dead tissue from the wound.
2. *Sharp Surgical Debridement*: This type of debridement is usually performed in the operating room by a

physician and includes the aggressive removal of large amounts of tissue (Stage IV pressure ulcers or burns), or life-threatening infection processes (necrotizing fasciitis) that require immediate removal.

3. *Laser Debridement*: This type of debridement applies a pulsed CO2 laser beam to cauterize severed vessels while leaving behind a sterilized wound bed. It is appropriate for split-thickness skin grafting in patients with burn injuries.

4. *Waterjet Hydrosurgery*: This type of sharp debridement ablates wound debris using a saline beam delivered via a small, highly powered pump and high-pressure tubing that produce a focused beam of up to 15,000 pounds per square inch (psi).

Advantages of Sharp Debridement

Sharp debridement is quick, may be combined with other debridement methods (thereby speeding up the process), and can be performed in a variety of settings.

Disadvantages of Sharp Debridement

The appropriateness of performing sharp debridement on patients who are receiving anticoagulant therapy or who have a current wound infection should be discussed with the physician. Considerations include: using caution to avoid introducing transient bacteremia from infected wounds; cost; the success of laser and waterjet debridement are highly dependent upon the clinician's skill; and delayed healing if adjacent healthy tissue is injured in the process.

Autolytic Debridement

Autolysis is considered selective debridement in that only the necrotic tissue is liquefied by the body's own enzymes while healthy tissue is spared. Wound fluid accumulates under semi occlusive or occlusive dressings. This fluid accumulation causes the body's own enzymes and moisture to rehydrate, soften, and liquefy eschar and/or slough. This debridement method is recommended for clean wounds with only a small amount of necrotic tissue. As the necrotic tissue dissolves and becomes gooey with discolored fluid, the wound bed will temporarily appear larger in size, but this does not mean that the dressing is infecting the wound. The extent of damage to the wound will start to become apparent as necrotic tissue is dissolved. Success of the debridement procedure should be clearly observable within 3 to 4 days. Autolytic debridement is a good choice when anticoagulant therapy renders surgical debridement unfeasible.

Advantages of Autolytic Debridement

Autolytic debridement can be used alone or in conjunction with other debridement techniques. It is safe, easy, the least painful approach, and relatively inexpensive.

Disadvantages of Autolytic Debridement

Autolysis is a slow process. It must be monitored very closely as it may promote anaerobic growth and infection, as well as for maceration. Skin protectant should be applied to periwound skin if drainage increases. The wound must be kept clean and the dressing changed according to the amount of drainage.

Enzymatic Debridement

Two types of enzymes are used to accelerate degradation and debridement in enzymatic debridement. They are categorized as:

- *Fibrinolytics:* Elase.
- *Collagenases:* Santyl.

Enzymes are prescribed by a physician and are available as topical ointments, creams, or sprays. The product can be applied directly to the wound or applied to gauze that is gently placed on specific tissue and covered as appropriate with a secondary dressing. Enzymatic debridement requires 1 to 3 dressing changes a day.

Enzymes are not as effective in dry environments and may require crosshatching the eschar. Crosshatching is done by using a scalpel to make shallow slits (like a tic-tac-toe frame) in the eschar. Do not penetrate through the eschar to avoid damaging the base of the wound under the eschar.

═════════════════════════════*FAST FACTS in a NUTSHELL*

Selective and Nonselective Enzymes

Read the product insert to determine if a product is selective or nonselective. Nonselective enzymes will harm surrounding healthy tissue. When using non-selective enzymes, it is important to apply a skin protectant to the surrounding skin.

Advantages of Enzymatic Debridement

It can be used alone or in conjunction with other debridement techniques; it is safe, easy, and minimally painful.

Disadvantages of Enzymatic Debridement

Costs can add up, depending upon the debridement area and how often dressings are changed. Prescription costs have reimbursement implications. Enzymatic debridement must be avoided with the use of heavy metal antimicrobials such as silver and zinc, which can deactivate the enzymatic process. Also, dark-colored ointments make accurate wound assessment difficult. At present, there is a lack of research regarding the ability of active ingredients in fibrinolytics (Elase) and collagenases (Santyl) to target specific necrotic tissue in wounds, making informed choices somewhat difficult.

FAST FACTS in a NUTSHELL

Elase and Santyl are options based on a facility's proto-col, formulary, availability, and cost. Even when a prod-uct insert states that the product is selective by nature, it must be monitored with good judgment. Enzymatic debriding products may damage healthy skin in com-promised patients, who already are at risk for impaired healing.

Biodebridement

Biodebridement consists of maggot therapy, which is FDA approved as a "'prescription only"' medical intervention. Sterile fly maggots are used to break down and ingest infected or necrotic tissue. Typically, about 10 maggots per square centimeter of necrotic tissue are used. The maggots are kept in the wound for 48 to 72 hours using a protective net dressing outlined with a hydrocolloid base.

Advantages of Biodebridement

The maggots do not damage healthy tissue. They work con-stantly, and after 72 hours, they can be destroyed.

Disadvantages of Biodebridement

In addition to the base cost of maggots, other cost factors include their containment mechanism, special dressings, and shipping. The maggots must be ordered, shipped, and used within 12 hours of receipt. Patient education is essen-tial in helping patients accept this helpful treatment inter-vention, as many patients fear that the maggots will escape from the protective dressing on the wound and end up in the bed with them. Patients also do not like the "creepy-crawly" feeling of maggots. There is a learning curve for successful outcomes, and the education process can be difficult at best for both the patient and the health care professional.

Chemical Debridement

The use of Dakin's solution, which denatures protein, is a method of chemical debridement that makes the wound slough and the wound eschar more easily removed. Dakin's solution is a dilution of 0.025% sodium hypochlorite, which is effective as an antimicrobial solution. The surrounding tissue must be protected with an appropriate skin barrier.

Advantages of Chemical Debridement

It is inexpensive, and it can be soaked in gauze and placed in large wounds and cavities. It is a beneficial initial treatment that is useful for controlling infection and odor until surgical debridement is performed.

Disadvantages of Chemical Debridement

The use of Dakin's solution is a short-term treatment and should not be used for more than 10 days because of its nonselective cytotoxicity. There is conflicting evidence about the ideal dilution. The container should be properly marked with the solution name and dilution amount.

Mechanical Debridement

Mechanical debridement is nonselective to the wound bed and edges of the wound, making it painful. The patient must be premedicated, and there must be ample time for the medication to take effect prior to the debridement procedure. Mechanical debridement methods include:

- Using scissors or forceps to lift and trim away loose eschar.
- Wet-to-dry dressings.
- Irrigation.
- Hydrotherapy.

Wet-to-Dry Dressings Done correctly, wet-to-dry dressings are painful and should be changed every 4 to 6 hours. The gauze is moistened with saline, allowed to dry in the wound, and then pulled off the wound along with the trapped debris.

Advantages: They are relatively inexpensive and simple to administer.

Disadvantages: Wetting the dressing before removing it (to alleviate pain) defeats the purpose of aggressively removing dead tissue, and packing the gauze too tightly will bruise the surrounding tissue. The frequency of dressing changes is time consuming. Also, airborne dispersal of bacteria is significant during the removal of the dry dressings.

Irrigation

This type of debridement is performed with equipment that combines a pulsating irrigation fluid with suction. This treatment usually takes 15–30 minutes and is performed twice daily at a pressure range from 4–15 psi.

- High-pressure irrigation delivers pressure of 8–12 psi; for example, a 35-mL syringe with a 19-gauge angiocatheter.
- Pulsatile high-pressure lavage provides intermittent high-pressure irrigation combined with suction. The pressure may be adjusted.

═══════════════════════════*FAST FACTS in a NUTSHELL*

A bulb syringe delivers a psi of only 4 (or less) and is not sufficient to remove eschar and slough from a wound bed. Check the effectiveness of your wound cleanser spray'. The psi should be noted on the bottle.

Advantages: It provides effective debridement and has been shown to improve granulation tissue growth.

Disadvantages: It has the potential for dissemination of bacteria from the spray. A mask, gloves, gown, and goggles must be worn by the wound care nurse, and the patient and others must be protected from the spray. Supplies may be costly and the process is time consuming. Its use should be avoided with patients on anticoagulant therapy.

Hydrotherapy

Hydrotherapy is cleaning by immersion, showering, or spraying. It is indicated for patients who need aggressive cleaning or softening of necrotic tissue (such as burn patients).

Advantages: It is an effective debridement method for large surface areas, the loosening of adherent necrotic tissue, and dressings.

Disadvantages: It may cause periwound maceration, put the patient at risk for water-borne infection, and increase cross-contamination among patients.

5

Documenting and Photographing Wounds

INTRODUCTION

""If you didn't document it, it didn't happen."

—Anonymous

A wound care nurse's documentation should provide information about thorough assessments, interventions, and patients" responses to wound care treatment. The wound care nurse should also document accurate and complete wound care evaluations, treatment modifications, and outcomes. Documentation serves as the round-the-clock communication tool for all members of the health care team. As a wound care nurse, your documentation is your legal defense, your verification of communication, your basis for treatment decisions, and your reasons for modifications. Documentation and photographs provide evidence. Moreover, the facility that you work for is paid based on accurate documentation.

In this chapter, you will learn:

1. How good documentation is based on national, local, and facility guidelines, standards of care, and protocols.
2. The types of photographic documentation.
3. About wound care documentation forms.

THE KEY TO GOOD DOCUMENTATION: BE THOROUGH AND CLEAR

Documentation Guidelines

Know where documentation guidelines originate.

The National Level

- *The American Medical Association (AMA):* A nurse practitioner who has a Medicare provider number and is billing Medicare under that number must follow the AMA guidelines (http://www.ama-assn.org).
- *The Center for Medicare and Medicaid Services (CMS):* Nurse practitioners and wound care specialists (members of the Wound, Ostomy and Continence Nurses Society [WOCN] and certified wound specialists [CWSs]) who do not bill Medicare directly for their professional services are required to provide the level of documentation required by the facility where they work (http://www.cms.gov).
- *The Agency for Healthcare Research and Quality (AHRQ* [formerly the Agency for Health Care Policy and Research (AHCPR)]: This agency promotes evidence-based practice by developing evidence reports through twelve evidence-based practice centers (EPCs). The topics range from common conditions to high-cost and high-volume conditions and significant clinical health care delivery (especially for Medicare and Medicaid populations). The AHRQ has become known as the science partner with private and public

facilities "in their efforts to improve the quality, effectiveness, and appropriateness of health care by synthesizing the evidence and facilitating the translation of evidence-based research findings" (http://www.ahrq.gov/clinic/epc).

The Local Level

- *The Medicare guidelines required by the facility for which you work:* Identify and follow these guidelines.
- *The Joint Commission (JC):* This organization assesses quality and safety in hospital facilities by setting standards and issuing accreditation to those facilities that meet these standards. If the JC finds any fault, the facility must make improvements within a set period of time or the facility could lose accreditation and even the right to be paid by Medicare.
  1. Know and understand the JC's *Do Not Use* Abbreviation List.
  2. Know and understand your facility's or organization's documentation protocols, policies, and/or guidelines, as the JC may ask to see them.
- *State Board of Nursing*
  1. Know and understand your State Board of Nursing wound care guidelines, such as Wound Debridement by Licensed Nurses and Patient Assessment.
  2. Know how to get in touch with your State Board of Nursing and have contact information available for the wound care team.
- *Your Facility's Wound Care Guidelines*
  1. Make sure that your facility has current wound care and documentation guidelines. Compare them with Medicare's, the JC's, and the State Board of Nursing's' guidelines.
  2. Remember to document the following:
     - Physician order(s).
     - The initial cause of and when the patient acquired the wound(s), including the date if possible.

- The initial evaluation, previous treatments, patient responses, and outcomes.
- Underlying conditions (e.g., diabetes) that may interfere with healing.
- Pain issues, medications, and psychosocial barriers.
- Skin assessment, routine care, and moisture management.
- Repositioning, turning schedules, and pressure-reducing bed/chair options.
- Nutritional status and labs.
- Wound assessment, characteristics, and plan.
- Treatments, description of instrument(s) used, and supplies.
- Treatment modifications related to changes in the patient's condition.
- Patient and/or family education and follow-up.
- Referrals related to nutrition, diabetes, smoking, vascular issues, podiatry, etc.
- Treatment time and signature.

PHOTOGRAPHIC DOCUMENTATION

Key Elements of Photograpic Documentation

- Obtain the patient's/resident's consent prior to taking photos.
- Provide good lighting and use the same camera, the same image resolution, and the same zoom setting each time a follow-up photo is obtained.
- Take each photo from the same angle, rotation, height, and distance.
- Use an ID label (name, date, patient number/code, location of the wound, and room number). This may be part of the wound measurement grid and should be placed alongside the wound before taking a photo.

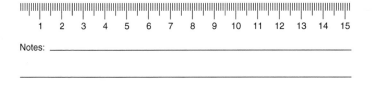

FIGURE 5.1   Example of a Wound Measurement Grid
Measured in centimeters (1 inch = 2.54 cm).

- Make sure that the wound position is the same each time a photo is obtained.
- Make sure that you wear approved protective gear (gloves, gown, and/or goggles) if you will appear in the photo.
- Consistently use photos to document each occurrence of pre- and post-debridement.
- Ensure that proper identification appears within the photo, not on the photo. This is a permanent part of the medical record. Do not write on the developed photo.
- Make sure that all photos are labeled consistently and stored in the same patient album and/or gallery.

Photographs of wounds can be the most reliable and accurate means of documentation if they are taken correctly. Photographs should be taken when the patient is first admitted and thereafter on a regular basis. Initial photographs provide a reference for monitoring the healing or deterioration of the skin/wound integrity.

Patient Name _____ Patient Number _____
Date _____ Rm # _____ Braden Score _____
Admit _____
Taken by _____ Physician _____
Location _____ Wound Type _____
Width (cm) _____ Length (cm) _____ Area (cm²) _____
Depth (cm) _____

Place Photo Here

Figure 5.2   Patient Photo Documentation Form

━━━━━━━━━━━━━━━━━*FAST FACTS in a NUTSHELL*

Types of Photographic Documentation Software

- The Polaroid HealthCam®II
- Savant Imaging
- Pixar®CDM

TABLE 5.1   Documentation Help Sheets

Braden Scale: Pressure Ulcers

Patient seen for low Braden score _____.

Patient has Stage _____, Location _____,

Measures _____.

Drainage (mild, moderate, heavy, serous,

serosanguinous, sanguinous).

Base is/has (granulation, slough, eschar, color).

Skin surrounding ulcer is (pink, intact, macerated).

Edges (well-defined, epiboly).

Cleaned with _____;

covered with

Risk factors such as incontinence, exposure to friction/sheer/

immobility/decreased sensation.

Skin intact over bony prominences with prevention strategies

in place.

Wound VAC

Date/time of dressing change.

Patient is premedicated per nurse.

Wound assessment: periwound skin, wound bed, odor,

presence of undermining and/or tunneling.

Wound cleaned with:

-Foam (black, white, silver) dressing applied to wound bed

sides, tunneling, and undermining.

-Transparent tape/drape placed and extended over foam

dressing by 3–5 cm.

-Clamps, tubing, and drapes checked for airtight seal.

Negative pressure running at _____mmHg.

Wound volume drainage in canister: small, moderate,

excessive.

Patient tolerated procedure _____

Continued

TABLE 5.1   Documentation Help Sheets *Continued*

Ostomy/Colostomy/
Urostomy
Stoma location and size: prolapse, ulceration, bulging.
Appearance (pink, red, necrosis, mucocutaneous separation).
Evidence of bleeding, infection.
Pouch type (one-piece or two-piece pouch).
Peristomal area:
Patient expresses positive behavior and proper techniques.
Output/type:

Trach
Small ulceration noted under trach plate, very difficult to
visualize due to placement. Foam dressing applied to help
with secretion absorption.

Articulating Words and Spelling

Achilles tendon	Gluteal fold
Agitation	Groin area
Buttocks	Incontinent
Cellulitis	Inflammation
Copious	Origin
Deterioration	Perineum
Diarrhea	Progression
DTI presents itself	Scrotum
Erythemia	Subsiding
Exacerbated	Unknown etiology
Fragile	Venous dermatitis
Generalized	First metatarsal

Defining the Spectrum of Simple to Complex Wounds

6

Skin Injuries

INTRODUCTION

A wound care nurse consultant was called to evaluate a "skin tear." Removal of the patient's gauze dressing revealed a jagged tear running the length of the forearm, a superficial hematoma extending from the wrist to the elbow, bruising of the surrounding skin, and edema of the hand. The consulting wound care nurse recommended immediate transfer of the patient to a hospital for X-rays to rule out fractures and for wound closure that resulted in 28 stitches. The staff was thankful for the consultation. A follow-up in-service was scheduled to review guidelines for evaluating skin injuries, skin damage, and skin tears.

In this chapter, you will learn:

1. The causes of and treatments for superficial skin injuries.
2. The difference between a deep tissue injury and a Stage I pressure ulcer.
3. How to classify and care for skin tears.

SUPERFICIAL SKIN INJURIES

Superficial skin injuries are wounds that are not related to "pressure" injuries (intensity of pressure, duration of pressure, or tissue tolerance). Therefore, superficial skin injuries are not documented under the National Pressure Ulcer Advisory Panel (NPUAP) as Stage I or II wounds. They are defined as superficial or partial thickness wounds. These skin injuries include abrasions, scrapes, tape burns, bruises, superficial burns, cuts, and scratches. They may be related to a disease process, trauma, medications, bites, or chemicals.

Abrasions, Scrapes, and Tape Burns

These superficial skin injuries are skin patches that have been scraped or peeled off.

Treatment

Remove the brush from an Ultradex E-Z scrub sponge and gently scrub with sponge to clean the area and remove dirt and debris. Apply Xeroform gauze and a dry sterile dressing.

Bruises

Sometimes called contusions, bruises are caused from a direct blow or a crushing injury that damages the blood vessels, causing bleeding in the dermis.

Treatment

If the injury happened recently, apply a cold compress.

Superficial Burns

Some examples of superficial burns include sunburns and minor scalds.

Treatment

Flush with cool water to stop the burning process. Remove the brush from an Ultradex E-Z scrub sponge. Gently cleanse the area. Apply a generous amount of skin protectant and reapply as needed.

Superficial Cuts and Scratches

Superficial cuts and scratches are cutting or slicing injuries to the top layer of skin (the epidermis) that do not penetrate the dermis. They may be contaminated with soil, feces, or saliva.

When in doubt, assume that superficial cuts and scratches are dirty.

Treatment

Remove the brush from an Ultradex E-Z scrub sponge and gently scrub to clean the area. Flush or irrigate with saline solution, and apply pressure if needed to stop bleeding. Apply antimicrobial ointment, bring the edges of the wound together, and secure them with a dressing.

FAST FACTS in a NUTSHELL

Three of the most common skin injuries that get confused in documentation are *contact dermatitis, denuded buttocks,* and *candidiasis.*

Contact Dermatitis

Occurs in an area where skin touches skin, such as underarms, skin folds, or buttocks. The excoriation is confined to an area, and may burn, sting, and/or itch.

Continued

Continued

Denuded Buttocks

Presents as reddened erosion from exposure to urine or stool, and may progress to vesicular blisters filled with clear or bloody fluid.

Candidiasis

Presents as a red, pustular fungal rash with a cheese-like odor. Within body folds, it is identified by its "cottage cheesy" secretion build up.

Treatment

For contact dermatitis and denuded buttocks: Gently cleanse the area, pat to dry, and then generously apply barrier paste. Generosity applying the paste will make it much less painful to remove.

For candidiasis: Absorb or prevent moisture by using wide-mesh gauze or towels between skin folds, air-drying (with or without) fan using a tent style cover for privacy, and clean often taking care not to spread. 'Burrow's solution soaks are soothing for burning and pruritus. Notify physician.

════════════════════════════*FAST FACTS in a NUTSHELL*

Ultradex E-Z scrub sponges contain chloroxylenol (PCMX), which is used as a mild antimicrobial soap. The sponges are effective in removing dirt and debris and are not as painful as other methods of cleansing.

DEEP TISSUE INJURIES AND PRESSURE ULCERS

The National Pressure Ulcer Advisory Panel (NPUAP) provides the following definitions:

- *Deep Tissue Injury (DTI)*: "Purple or maroon localized area of discolored intact skin or blood-filled blister due to damage of underlying soft tissue from pressure and/or shear."
- *Pressure Ulcer*: "Localized injury to the skin and/or underlying tissue usually over a bony prominence, as a result of pressure, or pressure in combination with shear and/or friction. A number of contributing or confounding factors are also associated with pressure ulcers."
  - *Stage I Pressure Ulcer*: "Intact skin with non-blanchable redness of a localized area usually over a bony prominence. Darkly pigmented skin may not have visible blanching; its color may differ from the surrounding area."

Both Stage I pressure ulcers and DTIs "may be preceded by tissue that is painful, firm, mushy, boggy, warmer or cooler as compared to adjacent tissue." It is clinically important to differentiate between a Stage I pressure ulcer and a DTI

Deep Tissue Injury (DTI)

Think of the etiology of a DTI as a high level of external pressure affecting the deep tissues at the bone–muscle interface. This pressure causes ischemia (cell death) at the muscle bed level. The superficial tissue near the skin surface rapidly becomes compromised from the injury and shear. The DTI becomes purple or maroon and then takes on the appearance of a blood-filled blister.

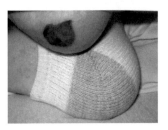

Stage I Pressure Ulcer

An early indication that a patient is at risk for a Stage I pressure ulcer is that erythema (redness) becomes white, or blanches, when pressure is applied with the fingertip. The redness quickly returns when pressure is released. If pressure is alleviated soon, blood flow will return.

Nonblanchable erythema over an intact bony prominence indicates impaired blood supply caused by the surface capillaries collapsing from an external intensity of pressure. Redness does not blanch and turn white with fingertip pressure.

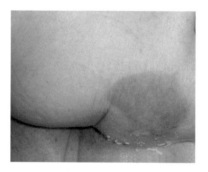

=FAST FACTS in a NUTSHELL

To prevent the development of a pressure ulcer, it is important to provide the following care:

- Turn the patient at least every 2 hours, and more frequently if needed.
- Each person's arterial and venous blood flow pressures vary and may cause a need for more frequent position changes. Check for blanching erythema.
- Use caution and care when turning a patient.
- Be gentle, as fragile skin bruises and tears easily.

Understanding the pathologic effect of pressure helps the nurse be aware of the causes of pressure intensity. Here are some key terms used to define how pressure is measured. By understanding these terms, the nurse is more aware if pressure the patient is experiencing is excessive or not.

Capillary closing pressure: Minimal amount of pressure required to collapse the capillary and occlude the blood flow (12–32 mmHg).

Muscle: Redistributes the pressure load.

Vascular circulation: Segmental (arterial vessels), perforator (supplies muscles and skin), and cutaneous (also thermoregulation).

The wound care nurse must understand and oversee the following factors that contribute to the' development of pressure ulcers:

- Pressure effects: Intensity of pressure, duration of pressure, and tissue tolerance.
- Off-loading and off-loading surfaces: See Chapter 15.
- Shear, friction, and nutritional debilitation.

Care and Prevention

- Apply barrier paste thick enough so that the top layer of the paste is removed with urine/stool.
- Re-apply after each episode; this is much less painful to patient.

SKIN TEARS

A skin tear is a wound resulting from trauma, which causes separation of the epidermis and dermis. Depending upon the severity of the friction and/or shearing forces, the tear can be a simple tear such as a rip around a fingerprinted bruise, or a severe tear consisting of flap loss, hematoma, and tissue death.

The Payne–Martin Classification System for Skin Tears

Category 1: The entire epidermal flap can be approximated.
A. Linear type, in which the epidermis and dermis are pulled in one layer from the supporting structure.
B. Flat type, in which the epidermis and dermis are separated, but the epidermis flap can be approximated to within 1 mm of the wound margins.
Category 2: There is a partial thickness loss of the flap.
A. Less than 25% of epidermal flap is lost.
B. More than 25% of the epidermal flap is lost.
Category 3: There is complete loss of the flap, causing a partial thickness wound.
There are two other classification systems for skin tears:

- Dunkin's (2003) Four-Category Classification of Pretibial Injuries
- Belson's (2008) Seven-Category Classification of Pretibial Injuries

No matter which classification system you choose to use, it is most important to document what you assess, especially if the injury is present upon admission of the patient.

Remember, documentation should include: pain level; date on which the trauma happened; cause of the trauma; location, size, and wound classification. Do not "stage" skin tears—they are not related to pressure.

Treatment Options for Skin Tears

- Remove the brush from an Ultradex E-Z scrub sponge and gently cleanse the area.
- For the remaining flap, gently flush or irrigate with saline solution or nontoxic wound cleanser, and pat dry. Apply pressure if needed to stop bleeding.
- Reposition and approximate the remaining flap.

- Choose the dressing based on the wound and drainage. Several optimal choices are silicone-faced foams, hydrogel sheets, and antimicrobial gels.
- Do not apply tension when applying the dressing.
- If you are using occlusive films, place an arrow on the dressing to indicate the direction of the skin flap. The arrow will indicate that the caretaker should remove the dressing in that direction and avoid pulling off the fragile flap.
- Carefully consider skin sealants or liquid barriers.
- Optimal secondary dressings are elastic net or tubular support dressings, ranging in size, as opposed to tape.

═══════════════════════════════*FAST FACTS in a NUTSHELL*

Recommended Tetanus Booster Protocol

- Minor, clean wounds: Obtain booster within 72 hours. Booster needed every 10 years.
- Dirty wounds: Obtain booster within 24 hours. Booster needed every 5 years.

Care and Prevention of Skin Tears

My favorite skin care quote is, "Lube and goob," and my least favorite is, "A little dab will do you." Educate the patient, family members, and the caretaker regarding frequent application of moisturizers, hydration, and protection alternatives.

- When choosing moisturizers, opt for pH-balanced, olive-based, alcohol-free protectants that contain silicones, if possible. They provide nourishment to the skin.
- If the patient is ambulatory, suggest that he or she keep moisturizer in the bathroom and apply every time he or she uses the bathroom.

- The caretaker may choose to remoisturize the patient each time oral care is performed, or to coincide with the turning schedule (a good routine practice).
- Use a lift sheet to move and/or turn the patient gently.
- Pad bedrails, wheelchair arms, and any other surfaces with which the skin tear comes in contact.
- Use pillows or blankets to support a restless patient and prevent the patient from dangling the arms and legs.

Time and tender loving care are unique, irreplaceable, and necessary resources of the wound care nurse. Helping colleagues and other staff understand this concept will help heal and lessen the incidence of skin injuries for patients and promote better health care.

7

Common Chronic Wounds

INTRODUCTION

Lower-extremity ulcers are the most common chronic wounds, with 80–90% of these wounds being related to chronic venous insufficiency (CVI). Cigarette smoking is the underlying cause of an estimated 40% of incidences of CVI in the United States, and the incidence of CVI is approximately equal at 20% for both men and women. Of the more than 4,000 toxic compounds contained in cigarette smoke, nicotine, carbon monoxide, and hydrogen cyanide are the most damaging to human tissue, causing vasoconstriction and tissue ischemia. Just one cigarette can trigger skin vasoconstriction for about 90 minutes. Is this a relevant coincidence or correlation? The cost of chronic wounds is a staggering $20 billion annually. This chapter will cover venous insufficiency, lymphedema, arterial and pressure ulcers (staged), and neuropathic/diabetic wounds.

In this chapter, you will learn:

1. Commonalities and characteristics related to the most common chronic wounds, including venous insufficiency ulcers, lymphedema, arterial ulcers, pressure ulcers, and diabetic ulcers.
2. Indications for established testing procedures to confirm pathology diagnoses.
3. Treatment and therapy priorities.

CHRONIC WOUNDS

Even though it has been said that all chronic wounds start out as acute wounds, the wound care nurse looks for a biological or physiological reason why a patient's wounds are not healing. Common characteristics of chronic wounds are loss of skin and tissue, lack of response to conventional types of treatments, unapproximated wound edges, and failure to move beyond the inflammatory phase of wound healing.

VENOUS INSUFFICIENCY ULCERS

Venous insufficiency ulcers are commonly called venous stasis ulcers.

Characteristics of Venous Ulcers

- *Location*: Medial malleolus (gaiter area).
- *Wound and wound edges*: Large and irregular.
- *Wound bed*: Ruddy red, possibly with yellow slough.
- *Volume of exudate*: Moderate to large amount.
- *Appearance of surrounding skin*: Depending upon the dressing and care, it could be macerated, crusted, and scaled; have a hemosiderin stain; be edematous; be hyperpigmented; and/or be characterized by lipodermatosclerosis.
- *Pain level*: Dull to severe, requiring medication before a dressing change.

Pathophysiology of Venus Insufficiency Ulcers

The venous system of the lower extremities is made up of deep veins, superficial veins, and perforator veins. They all have one-way valves that support the venous blood (against gravity) as it returns to the heart. The calf muscle and one-way valves work together to block backflow. You can think of the heart, calf muscle, and one-way valves as a faucet, the arteries and veins as a hose, and the blood as water. When you turn the faucet off and it (valves and calf muscles) does not work properly, the result is a constant drip effect, causing the blood to pool and leading to venous hypertension and ulcer formation.

Indications for Testing Procedures

Besides providing a correct diagnosis, the test results will identify obstructions, anatomic function, the vascular system involved, and/or other abnormalities contributing to a venous insufficiency ulcer. The results will provide the foundation for interventions, therapy, and treatment. The first signs of venous hypertension usually are leakage around the medial malleolus and the skin beginning to change from dark red or purple and itchy to painful and swollen. Generally, a physician will order a test if the wound care nurse provides a supportive rationale of the patient's need for it.

Testing Procedures

There is a wide variety of testing procedures from which to choose to assist in diagnosing venous insufficiency ulcers. These include:

- *Duplex Imaging:* It is noninvasive and is available with or without color images of anatomy and hemodynamic function.

- *Doppler Ultrasonography:* It is noninvasive; it is an ultrasound of pulse and allows calculation of the ankle-brachial index (ABI).
- *Photoplethysmography:* It is noninvasive and uses infrared light and a transducer probe to measure electrical impedance, venous reflux, and filling times.
- *Contrast Venography:* It is invasive; it produces a radiographic picture of the venous system, usually done before surgery.

Treatment and Therapy Priorities

The selection of treatment and therapy priorities depends upon the stage of prevention, management, or treatment of the venous insufficiency ulceration.

Prevention Stage

- The goal is to reduce pooling of blood and to prevent ulcers.
- Provide patient education about regular exercise and weight reduction, if indicated.
- Simple strategies to assist patients in getting regular exercise include:
  - If they sit or stand for long periods of time, they can exercise by extending and flexing the feet, ankles, and legs often.
  - When sitting or lying down, they can elevate the legs above the heart. Sitting in a recliner does not mean that the legs are above the heart.
- Encourage daily good skin hygiene (using soap, water, and lotion).
- Make sure that patients are compliant with wearing compression stockings. Forewarn patients that swelling hurts under compression, but after the swelling has gone down, the compression is much more tolerable and even desirable. Encourage patients to see this process through.

Management Stage

- The goal is to address CVI by improving venous return.
- Obtain a vascular consult for:
  - Surgical management: Possible vein ligation, phlebectomy, or vein bypass.
  - Nonsurgical treatment: Sclerotherapy or endovenous thermal ablation.

Treatment Stage

- The goal for treating a venous ulcer is to determine what the wound needs.
- Providing pain control, infection control, and debridement are fundamental.
- Consider using an antimicrobial dressing based on the amount of drainage and depth of the wound. Avoid tape. Excellent secondary dressings are elastic net dressings that may be sized and customized as garment dressings, allowing maximum airflow.
- Use a protectant lotion or barrier on surrounding skin for prevention of maceration.

Types of Compression Therapy

- *Support Stockings:* Static short stretch; custom fit; vary in degrees of compression; difficult to apply but the patient/caregiver can learn to apply. (Example: Biersdorf-jobst)
- *Orthotic Device:* Static inelastic; must be premeasured; custom fit; easy to apply or take off for wound assessment; Velcro closures; bulky. (Example: Circ-Aid)
- *Zinc Paste Bandage:* Static inelastic; combined dressing and compression in one; soothing; does not stretch back with pressure changes; not a good choice for heavily draining wounds. (Examples: Unna Boot, Dome paste bandage)
- *Four-Layer System:* Static and inelastic layers; may be used for heavily draining wounds and adjusted to leg

shapes; maintains pressure for up to 1 week. (Examples: Profore, Dynaflex)
- *Limited-Stretch Wraps:* Static–elastic; has marks that indicate the correct degree of stretch; can be washed and reused. (Examples: Comprilan, Setopress)
- *Compression Pumps:* Dynamic; atrioventricular (AV) compression is safe for patients with arterial ischemia; can be used in the home, but patient is immobile for 2–4 hours; there is a rental charge. (Examples: AV Impulse, Intermittent Pneumatic Compression, Sequential Compression)

The common therapeutic compression level is 30–40 mmHg at the ankle; however, the physician may recommend a lower or higher level depending upon the patient's needs.

LYMPHEDEMA FLUID LEAKING

You can think of the lymphatic system as the traffic control police for plasma; their job is to remove toxins, pathogens, and malignant cells. If the lymphatic micropolice go on strike, then the fluid accumulates in distal areas, such as the hand or foot, and works its way up the limb as nonpitting edema. Eventually, the elasticity of the skin is destroyed; the skin thickens and becomes severely distorted. At this point, the condition is known as elephantiasis.

- Primary Elephantiasis: Inherited.
- Secondary Elephantiasis: Injury to lymphatic vessels.

The Common Stages of Lymphedema

- *Stage 0 (Latent):* Lymphedema is not present even though lymphatic vessels have been damaged.
- *Stage 1 (Spontaneously Reversible):* Tissue shows pitting with daily stress, but this reverses with rest.

- *Stage 2 (Spontaneously Irreversible):* Tissue is spongy, nonpitting, and bounces back, related to fibrosis formation.
- *Stage 3 (Lymphostatic Elephantiasis):* Tissue is hard, fibrotic, and unresponsive; swelling is irreversible and limbs are gigantic.

===============*FAST FACTS in a NUTSHELL*

Widely Accepted Testing Procedures for Lymphedema

Limb Circumference: Use the 2-cm rule: A– difference in circumference of 2 cm on either limb is significant.

Tissue Fluid Analysis: A protein content of between 1.0 and 5.5 g/dL is usually indicative of lymphedema, whereas 0.1 to 0.9 g/dL is more consistent with venous or cardiac edema.

Testing for Stemmer's Sign: Gently pinch and lift the skin at the base of the second toe (next to big toe). A test result is positive if the skin cannot be lifted.

Severity Grades for Lymphodema (Referenced to a Healthy Extremity)

- *Grade 1 (Mild Edema):* For hands, feet, and lower limbs, the difference in circumference is less than 4 cm.
- *Grade 2 (Moderate Edema):* For the entire limb, the difference in circumference is more than 4 cm, but less than 6 cm.
- *Grade 3a (Severe Edema):* For the entire limb and associated trunk quadrant, the difference in circumference is more than 6 cm.
- *Grade 3b (Massive Edema):* Same as Grade 3a except that two or more extremities are affected.
- *Grade 4 (Gigantic Edema):* Elephantiasis; head and face may be affected.

Magnetic resonance imaging (MRI) can rule out other causes of swelling.

Treatment and Therapy Priorities

The severity of the edema and the degree of fibrosis must be determined. Patients with venous insufficiency require 30–40 mmHg of compression. Lymphedema patients require more: 50–60 mmHg of compression.

The following treatments done in combination or individually are the most common:

- *Manual Lymph Drainage (MLD):* Facilitates contraction of smooth muscles in lymph vessels, helping to move the lymph fluid toward the heart.
  - Basic MLD and Full Complete Decongestive Therapy (CDT) Certification Information: http://www.norton school.com/lymphedemacourse.html
- *Intermittent Sequential Gradient Pump:* Helps break up fibrotic hard tissue.
- *Compression Wrapping:* Has 3 to 4 layers and has to be changed only once a week (depending upon the drainage level); enhances pumping action and resistance of lymph vessels. (Examples: Profore, Dynaflex)

Four-Layer Compression System Instructions

Incorporate practice in regular in-services, having nurses practice applications on each other. This practice will help prevent intimidation and improper applications.

- Follow appropriate wound care practice: Make sure skin is clean, dry, moisturized, and protected.
- Layer 1 provides a layer of padding for protection and absorbency. Do a spiral wrap with 50% overlap, beginning at the top of the toes, and ending right below the knee. Use cast batting or orthopedic wool.

- Layer 2 simply provides more padding. Do a spiral wrap with 50% overlap. Use a light-conforming bandage (unstretched). This is the layer omitted in three-layer compression.
- Layer 3 provides subbandage pressure. Wrap with a figure-eight technique, applying 50% extension as you wrap and using a 50% overlap. Use an Ace, long-stretch bandage.
- Layer 4 provides (along with layer 3) approximately 35–40 mmHg subbandage pressure. Do a spiral wrap with 50% overlap. Use an elastic cohesive bandage.
- Compression garments—custom fit or over-the-counter—should be worn by the patient daily for edema reduction and to re-establish a normal blood flow in the tissues. (Examples: Jobst, Juzo, Sigvaris, Solidea, Truform)

≡ *FAST FACTS in a NUTSHELL*

Tips for Compression Systems

Be aware of a risk for latex allergy if the compression system is not latex free.

Change the system every 5 to 7 days—or when drainage seeps through.

Depending upon the size of the leg, more packages of each dressing layer may be needed to maintain proper overlap. Don't skimp.

ARTERIAL ULCERS

Arterial ulcers are also known as ischemic ulcers.

Characteristics of Arterial Ulcers

- *Location*: The most distal points, including the toes, ankle, and top of feet (dorsum area).

- *Wound and Wound Edges:* Small, round, and with well-defined edges.
- *Wound Bed:* Pale, dry base, and black eschar.
- *Volume of Exudate:* Dry unless the wound is infected.
- *Appearance of Surrounding Skin:* Shiny skin with loss of hair and thick nails.
- *Pain Level:* Very painful, medication is necessary before a dressing change.

Ischemic arterial ulcers are caused by decreased blood flow to the lower extremities. Recall the faucet and water hose analogy for venous insufficiency ulcers. The heart, calf muscle, and one-way valves are the faucet, the arteries and veins are the hose, and the blood is the water. This analogy also applies to ischemic arterial ulcers, except that when the faucet is turned on, there is no water (i.e., blood carrying oxygen and nutrients), which leads to tissue ischemia.

Indications for Testing Procedures of Ischemic Pain

- *Intermittent Claudication:* Cramping pain and burning in calf muscle that occurs with physical activity but is relieved within 2–5 minutes of rest.
- *Nocturnal Pain:* Cramping pain that occurs when lying down from the leg being elevated and the heart slowing down.
- *Rest Pain:* Constant, deep, aching pain that is associated with forefoot, ankles, and toes when the legs are in a dependent position. Look for signs of "hanging foot."

Testing Procedures for Arterial Ulcers

- *Capillary Refill:* Normal refill time is less than 3 seconds when the toe pad is pressed.
- *Skin Temperature:* Compare one leg to the other to note any difference in temperature.
- *Ankle-Brachial Index (ABI):* Compares perfusion pressure of the lower limb to the upper arm.

- *Pulse Volume Recordings (PVRs):* Measure the changes in leg volume per heartbeat.
- *Doppler Waveforms:* Measure recoil of the artery, loss of elastic recoil of the artery, and occlusion or stenosis.
- *Lower-Extremity Arterial Study (LEA):* Known as the "super ABI," it pinpoints the exact location of blockage.
- *Transcutaneous Oxygen (TcpO2):* Must be greater than 30 mmHg to perform safe debridement. If TcpO2 is less than 20 mmHg, the wound/ulcer will not heal.

Guidelines for Obtaining an ABI (Known as the Sixth Vital Sign)

You will need a blood pressure cuff and a Doppler system.

- Place the patient in a supine position and take his or her brachial systolic blood pressure in both arms. Use the higher systolic pressure.
- Place the blood pressure cuff on the affected leg, just above the malleoli.
- Place the Doppler probe at a 45-degree° angle, at the dorsalis pedis or posterior tibial artery.
- Inflate the cuff until there is no Doppler signal.
- Deflate the cuff until the Doppler signal returns. The point at which you hear the Doppler return is the systolic ankle pressure.
- Divide the ankle pressure by the systolic pressure to obtain the ABI.

Interpretation of an ABI

- 0.95 to 1.3: Normal range.
- 0.90 to 0.80: Moderate disease; patient may not show symptoms; can use compression.
- 0.80 to 0.50: Severe disease associated with claudication.
- Less than 0.50: Rest pain or gangrene.
- Unreliable: Diabetes.

Note: The ABI procedure can be billed if a physician reads it. An ABI is the initial screening for a vascular consult. A wound care nurse understands the importance of a vascular referral consult. Many amputations could be prevented by a timely vascular referral.

FAST FACTS in a NUTSHELL

Referral Criteria for a Patient to See a Vascular Physician: Routine, Semi-Urgent, or Urgent

- ABI:
  - Over 0.8: Routine referral.
  - Between 0.8 and 0.5: Semi-urgent referral.
  - Under 0.5: Urgent referral.
  - Under 1.0 with diminished or absent pulses: Semi-urgent referral.
- Gangrene present: Urgent referral, especially if gangrene is wet.
- Exposed bone or tendon: Urgent referral.
- Gross infection or cellulitis: Urgent referral.
- Nonhealing wounds despite 3+ pulses: Semi-urgent referral.

With grateful acknowledgment of Dr. Gregory Patterson, FACS, FASA. FAPWCA, FCCWS of Thomasville, Georgia for having taught me this.

Treatment and Therapy Priorities for Arterial Ulcers

Prevention Stage

The goal is to increase the circulation and perfusion to the ischemic area.

- Educate.
- Encourage the patient to exercise regularly.
- Encourage the patient to quit smoking.
- Encourage the patient to control his or her weight.
- Encourage the patient to maintain hydration.
- Encourage the patient to control and maintain normal blood glucose, serum cholesterol, and blood pressure.

Management Stage

The goal for arterial ulcers is to address peripheral arterial disease (PAD) by correcting the underlying arterial ischemia.

- Obtain a vascular consult for:
  - Surgical management: Angioplasty, stent, atherectomy, or surgery.
  - Nonsurgical treatment: Hyperbaric oxygen therapy or pharmacologic options.

Treatment Stage

The goal is to determine the wound care need and to deliver appropriate treatment.

- Control pain and infection.
- If there is dry gangrene with no signs of infection, paint the wound with 10% povidone-iodine solution, allow to dry, and wrap with dry gauze for protection.
- Ischemic wounds are not likely to show an inflammatory response. If changes to the wound are noted, seek a prompt vascular consult.
- Apply nongreasy protectant lotion to the surrounding skin to prevent cracking, itching, flaking, scaling, or peeling skin that could lead to infection.
- Consider an antimicrobial dressing based on the amount of drainage and depth of the wound. Avoid tape. Excellent secondary dressings are elastic net dressings, which may be sized and customized as secondary garment dressings, allowing maximum airflow.

PRESSURE ULCERS

Pressure ulcers, also known as pressure sores and bed sores, are on everyone's radar for the reasons outlined in the following. This information is very important to wound care nurses, as most pressure ulcers have been classified as preventable and their treatment is no longer reimbursed.

- In 2006, the AHRQ reported that nearly 9 of every 10 hospital stays involving pressure ulcers were covered by government health programs (Medicare and Medicaid). The cost for treatment of pressure ulcers averaged $37,800.
- In the AHRQ's *News and Numbers* report, patients that developed pressure ulcers before or after being hospitalized increased by almost 80% between 1993 and 2006.
- The Healthcase Cost and Utilization Program (HCUP) analysis was a 2008 statistical report of 503,300 nationwide pressure ulcer-related hospitalizations. The report found that pressure ulcers were a secondary diagnosis, meaning that they were acquired in hospitals, in 457,800 of these hospital admissions. Also, the death rate was about 1 in 8 for hospital-acquired pressure ulcers.
- Overall, hospital stays average 5 days and cost about $10,000. The HCUP analysis found that pressure ulcers extended hospital stays for 13 to 14 days and boosted costs between $16,755 and $20,430. Finally, the cost of adult hospital stays with a diagnosis of pressure ulcers in 2006 totaled $11.0 billion.

What these data mean to you and your facility is this: If a patient develops a hospital-acquired complication (HAC) such as a pressure ulcer, it will be tagged with an ICD-9-CM code, meaning that the patient has developed complicating conditions that necessitate increased payments. However, because of the Social Security Act 1886(d)(4)(D) that was passed in 2005, the increased reimbursement will be denied. The three criteria for designating an HAC were high cost, high volume, and a condition that could reasonably have been prevented through the application of evidence-based guidelines. Pressure ulcers, which are HACs, damage the reputation of everyone associated with the care of patients who develop them. Therefore, accurate knowledge and strategies for preventing and treating pressure ulcers are essential.

Pressure Ulcers Defined

Pressure ulcers are caused by unrelieved pressure on skin over bony prominences. Be aware of the three types of pressure that can lead to the development of a pressure ulcer:

1. *Pressure Intensity:* Pressure that is being applied externally to the skin.
   - *Capillary Pressure:* The force of fluid passing through (and keeping open) capillary membrane walls.
   - *Capillary Closing Pressure:* The minimal amount of pressure required to collapse a capillary. Standard capillary closing pressure is 12–32 mmHg.
2. *Pressure Duration:* Low pressure applied to the skin over a long period of time versus high pressure over a short period of time.
3. *Tissue Tolerance:* The capability of the tissue and the general condition of the skin and its supporting structures to endure the effects of pressure without damage.

The National Pressure Ulcer Advisory Panel (NPUAP) classifies pressure ulcers into four stages:

Stage I: Intact skin with nonblanchable redness; darkly pigmented skin may not have visible blanching; may be painful, firm, soft, and/or warmer or cooler as compared to adjacent tissue.

Stage II: May present as being superficial with separation or loss of epidermis, such as a blister or abrasion, or may present as partial thickness loss of dermis, such as a shallow, red or pink crater. *Note:* This stage should not be used to describe skin tears, tape burns, perineal dermatitis, maceration, or excoriation. Bruising indicates possible deep tissue injury.

Stage III: Full thickness skin loss involving damage to or necrosis of subcutaneous tissue that may extend down to, but not through, underlying fascia. The ulcer presents clinically as a deep crater with or without undermining of adjacent tissue. A small amount of slough may be present.

Stage IV: Full thickness skin loss with extensive destruction, tissue necrosis, or damage to muscle, bone, or supporting structures such as tendons or joint capsules. Undermining and sinus tracts also may be associated with Stage IV pressure ulcers.

Relieve or Reduce Pressure by:
- Using support surfaces designed to reduce pressure, including special beds, mattresses, and overlays.
- Do a "hand check."
  Slide your hand under the support surface under the pressure-point area.
  About 1 inch or more of support surface padding should be between your hand and the patient.
- Position the patient so that he or she is not lying or sitting on the pressure ulcer.
- Use pillows, blankets, or foam pads to alleviate pressure on knees, ankles, and heels.
- Change the patient's position at least every 2 hours or more if necessary.
- Place the patient in a 30-degree side-lying position and don't raise the head of the bed more than 30-degrees if possible.
- Do not use a donut cushion.
- When the patient is sitting, he or she should use good posture, keep the tops of the thighs horizontal, and not flex or extend ankles.

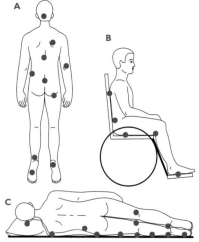

Dots show pressure points when lying on back (A),
when sitting (B), and when lying on side (C).

FIGURE 7.1   Pressure Relief Points

Used with permission from the NPUAP.
Predicting Pressure Ulcer Risk

Risk assessment forms should be initiated upon admission and repeated per facility protocol. ,Risk assessment tools are used to identify patients at risk, the level of risk, and the type of risk so that intervention can be started early, when patients are at a mild or moderate level of risk.

The most commonly used pressure ulcer assessment scale is the Braden scale.

Taking the Confusion Out of Reverse Staging

The NPUAP has issued a position statement regarding reverse staging and recommendations that include the following:

- Reverse staging should never be used to describe healing pressure ulcers related to the anatomical and structural layers of lost muscle, subcutaneous fat, and dermis. These tissues are replaced only as scar tissue.
- The maximum anatomic depth of tissue loss, once staged a III or IV, remains classified at that stage, for example, a healing Stage III or a healed Stage IV.
- The progression of healing pressure ulcers should be documented by characteristics such as size, depth, necrotic tissue, amount of exudate, etc.
- The NPUAP recognizes federal regulations requiring long-term care facilities to reverse staging. The Outcome and Assessment Information Set (OASIS) regulations will be discussed later.
- If a healed pressure ulcer reopens in the same anatomical site, the ulcer resumes the previous staging diagnosis.
- The NPUAP developed and validated the Pressure Ulcer Scale for Healing (PUSH, see Figure 7.3), a great tool to use in conjunction with OASIS assessment forms.

	1. Completely Limited	2. Very Limited	3. Slightly Limited	4. No Impairment
SENSORY PERCEPTION Ability to respond meaningfully to pressure-related discomfort	Unresponsive (does not moan, flinch, or grasp) to painful stimuli, due to diminished level of consciousness or sedation OR limited ability to feel pain over most of body.	Responds only to painful stimuli. Cannot communicate discorrfort except by moaning or restlessness OR has a sensory impairment which limits the ability to feel pain or discomfort over 1/2 of body.	Responds to verbal commands, but cannot always communicate discomfort or the need to be turned. OR has some sensory impairment which limits ability to feel pain or discomfort in 1 or 2 extremities.	Responds to verbal commands. Has no sensory deficit which would limit ability to feel or voice pain or discomfort.
MOISTURE Degree to which skin is exposed to moisture	**1. Constantly Moist** Skin is kept moist almost constantly by perspiration, urine. etc Dampness is detected every time patient is moved or turned.	**2. Very Moist** Skin is often but not always moist. Linen must be changed at least once a shift.	**3. Occasionally Moist:** Skin is occasionally moist, requiring an extra linen change approximately once a day.	**4. Rarely Moist** Skin is usually dry, linen only requires changing at routine intervals

94

| ACTIVITY
Degree of
physical activity | 1. Bedfast
Confined to bed. | 2. Chairfast
Ability to walk severely limited or nonexistent. Cannot bear own weight and/or must be assisted into chair or wheelchair. | 3. Walks Occasionally
Walks occasionally during day, but for very short distances, with or without assistance. Spends majority of each shift in bed or chair | 4. Walks Frequently
Walks outside room at least twice a day and inside room at least once every two hours during waking hours. |
| MOBILITY
Abilty to change and control body position | 1. Completely Immobile
Does not make even slight changes in body or extremity position without assistance. | 2. Very Limited
Makes occasional slight changes in body or extremity position but unable to make frequent or significant changes independentty. | 3. Slightly Limited
Makes frequent though slight changes in body or extremity position independently. | 4. No Limitation
Makes major and frequent changes in position without assistance. |

FIGURE 7.2   The Braden Scale for Predicting Pressure-Sore Risk   *Continued*

NUTRITION Usual food intake pattern	1. Very Poor	2. Probably Inadequate	3. Adequate	4. Excellent
	Never eats a complete meal. Rarely eats more than 1/2 of any food offered. Eats 2 servings or less of protein (meat or dairy products) per day. Takes fluids poorly. Does not take a liquid dietary supplement OR is NPO and/or maintained on liquids or IVs for more than 5 days.	Rarely eats a complete meal and generally eats only about 1/2 of any food offered. Protein intake includes only 3 servings of meat or dairy products per day. Occasionally will take a dietary supplement OR receives less than optimum amount of liquid diet tube feeding.	Eats over half of most meals. Eats a total of 4 servings of protein (meat, dairy products) per day. Occasionally will refuse a meal, but will usualy take a supplement when offered OR Is on a tube feeding or TPN regimen which probably meets most of nutritionai needs	Eats most of every meal. Never refuses a meal. Usually eats a total of 4 or more seivings of meat and dairy products. Occasionally eats between meals. Does not require supplementation.

FRICTION & SHEAR	1. Problem	2. Potential Problem	3. No Apparent Problem
	Requires moderate to maximum assistance in moving. Complete lifting without sliding against sheets is impossible. Frequently slides down in bed or chair, requiring frequent repositioning with maximum assistance. Spasticity, contractures or agitation lead to almost constant friction.	Moves feebly or requires minimum assistance. During a move, probably slides to some extent against sheets, chair, restraints or other devices. Maintains relatively good position in chair or bed most of the time but occasionally slides down.	Moves in bed and in chair independently and has sufficient muscle strength to lift completely during move. Maintains good position in bed or chair.

FIGURE 7.2 The Braden Scale for Predicting Pressure-Sore Risk

Source: Braden, B., & Bergstrom, N. Copyright 1988. Reprinted with permission. Permission should be sought to use this tool at www.bradenscale.com. Other services and products related to the Braden Scale are available to users free of charge at this site.

PUSH TOOL 3.0
(Pressure Ulcer Scale for Healing Tool 3.0)

Patient Name: Patient ID#:
Ulcer Location: Date:

DIRECTIONS:
Observe and measure the pressure ulcer according to the steps below. A comparison of total scores measured over time provides an indication of the improvement or deterioration in pressure ulcer healing. r——

		Subscore
Length x Width In cm2	0 1 2 3 4 5 6 7 8 9 10	
	0 1 2 3 4 5 6 7 8 9 10 0 <0.3 0.3-0.6 0.7-1.0 1.1-2.0 2.1-3.0 3.1-4.0 4.1-8.0 8.1-12.0 12.1-24.0 >24.0	
Exudate Amount	0 None 1 Light 2 Moderate 3 Heavy	
Tissue Type	0 Closed 1 Epithelial Tissue 2 Granulation Tissue 3 Slough 4 Necrotic Tissue	
Total Score =		

Step 1. Length x Width: Measure the greatest length (head to toe) and the greatest width (side to side) using a centimeter ruler. Multiply these two measurements (length x width) to obtain an estimate of surface area in square centimeters (cm²). Then select the corre¬sponding category for size on the scale and record the score. For example, a surface area of 3.0 cm² is scored 5. Caveat: Do not guess! Always use a centimeter ruler and always use the same method each time the ulcer is measured.

Step 2. Exudate Amount: Estimate the amount of exudate (drainage) present after removal of the dressing and before applying any topical agent to the ulcer. Estimate the exudate (drainage) as none, light, moderate, or heavy. Select the corresponding category for amount and record the score.

Step 3. Tissue Type: This refers to the types of tissue that are present in the wound (ulcer) bed. Score as a "4" if there is any necrotic tissue present. Score as a "3" if there is any amount of slough present and necrotic tissue is absent. Score as a "2" if the wound is clean and contains granulation tissue. A superficial wound that is reepithelial-izing is scored as a "1". When the wound is closed, score as a "0".

FIGURE 7.3   Push Tool 3.0

4 - Necrotic Tissue (Eschar): black, brown, or tan: tissue that adheres firmly to the wound bed or ulcer edges and may be either firmer or softer than surrounding skin.

3 - Slough: yellow or white tissue that adheres to the ulcer bed in strings or thick clumps, or is mucinous.

2 - Granulation Tissue: pink or beefy red tissue with a shiny, moist, granular appearance.

1 - Epithelial Tissue: for superficial ulcers, new pink or shiny tissue (skin) that grows in from the edges or as islands on the ulcer surface.

0 - Closed/Resurfaced: the wound is completely covered with epithelium (new skin).

Step 4: Sum the scores on the three elements of the tool to derive a total PUSH Score.

Step 5: Transfer the total score to the Pressure Ulcer Healing Graph. Changes in the score over time provide an indication of the changing status of the ulcer. If the score goes down, the wound is healing. If it gets larger, the wound is deteriorating.

FIGURE 7.3   Push Tool 3.0

Staging pressure ulcers is a classification method first designed by Dr. Darrell Shea, modified by the NPUAP, and adopted by the ACER Pressure Ulcer Guidelines Panels. Pressure ulcer staging is only appropriate for defining the maximum depth of tissue involvement.

The PUSH tool was developed by the NPUAP to monitor changes in pressure ulcers. NPUAP recommends using the tool at least weekly and if the condition of the patient or wound deteriorates. The three critical parameters used by the PUSH tool to score changes are: surface area, exudate amount, and tissue appearance. An increase in a score indicates wound deterioration and necessitates evaluation and possible treatment change.

Treatment and Therapy Priorities

Managing pressure ulcers should be a team approach to formulate a plan of care consistent with the patient's and family members' preferences, goals, and abilities.

- Eliminate the source of pressure and manage the tissue load (perpendicular force). Address the three major factors contributing to pressure ulcer development: shear, friction, and nutritional debilitation.
  - Consider and address pressure-relieving devices such as low-air-loss beds for patients who are unable to turn, have tissue breakdown, and need continuous blood flow to tissues.
  - Initiate a turning schedule that is ensured with documentation.
  - Protect a pressure ulcer with positioning devices, and limit sitting time and head elevation time.
  - Use lifting devices and bariatric equipment as needed.
  - Avoid donut cushions and sheepskin.
  - Chair-bound patients should reposition themselves every 15 minutes.
- Optimize the microenvironment with infection control and nutritional support.
  - Be attentive to nutritional assessments and laboratory parameters.
  - Be vigilant with sharp debridement regarding the potential for infection.
- Evaluate the wound repair and provide appropriate treatment. As a wound and/or a patient's needs change, so does the treatment plan. Remember that "One size (or one dressing) fits all" does not apply in wound care.
- Education is fundamental to quality improvement of pressure ulcer care and prevention. The National Pressure Ulcer Advisory Panel provides a variety of resources, education tools, and research provides information about many services, tools, experts in the field, and evidence-based practice regarding appropriate intervention for pressure ulcers.

DIABETIC ULCERS

The incidences of diabetes diagnoses are increasing in staggering numbers: The estimated annual treatment cost of diabetes alone in 2002 was $132 billion. The Centers for Disease Control and Prevention estimates that 23.6 million Americans currently have diabetes, and diabetes is the single most common cause of all amputations in the United States. Let's stop right here and contemplate amputation. Before there is amputation, there was an ulcer. Before there was an ulcer, there was neuropathy. What if prevention were a paramount, precedence priority with the loss of sensation and neuropathy? How many lower-extremity amputations (LEA's) could be prevented? Studies show that patient education and improved care diminish recidivism with diabetes.

Diabetic Neuropathy Origins

Nerve disorders caused by diabetes are called neuropathies and are thought to be caused by hyperglycemia and micro vascular disease. Nerve damage may be caused by other factors, such as mechanical injuries (e.g., carpal tunnel syndrome), lifestyle factors (e.g., smoking or alcohol use), and autoimmune factors that cause inflammation in nerves.

Hyperglycemia Slows Wound Healing

- It affects all stages of wound healing.
- It causes abnormal cell function; blood is more viscous.
- It impairs host defenses, leading to a higher risk of infection.
- It causes vascular disease, a catabolic state, and tissue hypoxia.
- It causes protein breakdown and diminished collagen synthesis.

==*FAST FACTS in a NUTSHELL*

Diabetic Testing

- Blood glucose must be controlled to under 200 mg/dL to attain a good surgical outcome.
- Glycosylated hemoglobin (A1c) should be less than 7.
- The Hemoglobin A1c Test shows the average blood glucose over a period of 2 to 3 months.

Types of Neuropathy

Sensory/Peripheral Neuropathy: Affects arms, legs, feet, and hands.

- *Signs:* Paresthesia (tingling, burning, prickling sensations), insensitivity to pain or temperature, loss of balance and coordination, and loss of deep tendon reflex.

Autonomic Neuropathy: Affects nerves in the heart (blood pressure) and internal organs.

- *Signs*: Anhidrosis (inability to sweat), hypoglycemia unawareness, and orthostatic hypotension.

Motor Neuropathy: Affects nerves controlling the muscles and results in muscle atrophy of the feet.

- *History:* Alcoholism, obesity, smoking, Raynaud's disease, hypertension, and heredity.

Routine Assessment

The Semmes–Weinstein microfilament test uses a 5.07 g monofilament that bends with 10 g of pressure.

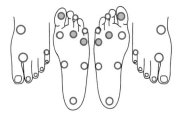

Directions
1. Touch the filament to the skin for 1 to 2 seconds, pushing hard enough to buckle the filament.
2. Place a √ in the circles where the patient feels the filament and an X in circles where sensation is not present.
3. Do not test over calluses, cracks, or the ulcer site.

FIGURE 7.4   Semmes–Weinstein Monofilament Test

Source: Courtesy of Health Resources and Services Administration (HRSA), www.hrsa.gov/leap/levelonescreening.htm

═══════════════════════════*FAST FACTS in a NUTSHELL*

Paperboard-handle monofilaments are affordable and practical. You can order monofilaments online at the following sites:

- http://medicalmonofilament.com
- http://www.medline.com

Wagner Classification of Diabetic Foot Ulcers

Diabetic ulcers are not pressure ulcers and should not be staged. The most commonly used scale for classifying diabetic ulcers is the Wagner Classification Scale, which grades ulcers based on appearance and depth.

TABLE 7.1	Wagner Classification Scale
Grade	Appearance, Location, and Depth of Ulcer
Grade 0	Pre-ulcerative lesion, healed ulcers, presence of bony deformity.
Grade 1	Superficial ulcer without subcutaneous tissue involvement.
Grade 2	Penetration through the subcutaneous tissue (may expose bone, tendon, ligament or joint capsule).
Grade 3	Osteitis, abscess, or osteomyelitis.
Grade 4	Gangrene of the forefoot.
Grade 5	Gangrene of the entire foot.

FAST FACTS in a NUTSHELL

Terminology for Documenting Common Diabetic Pressure Point Anatomical Sites

- Pes planus (flat foot)
- Dorsal and distal toes (bunionettes)
- Cocked-up toes (claw toes) from muscle atrophy
- Interdigital (superficial ulcers from nails related to toes curling medially)
- Corns (caused by pressure and friction from adjacent toe bones)
- Hallux valgus (one toe overrides or crosses completely over another one)
- Metatarsal head ulcers
- Heel cracks, hemorrhagic calluses, ingrown nails (onychocryptosis)
- Third metatarsal head exposure (a sign of osteomyelitis)

Treatment and Therapy Priorities for Diabetic Wounds

Diabetic wound priorities are education for compliance, glucose/glycemic control, prevention of amputation, vascular consult if needed, and wound care (debridement and infection control).

Off-loading therapy helps eliminate abnormal pressure points and protects the foot from ulcer formation or recurrence. There are a variety of off-loading options. Consider the patient's age, strength, environment, and daily activities. Be aware of complications (e.g., osteomyelitis, gangrene, or cellulitis), and quickly intervene with an aggressive treatment plan if needed. Remember that the priority goal is to prevent an ulcer and amputation.

═══════════════════════════════*FAST FACTS in a NUTSHELL*

Options for the Use of Off-Loading Therapy

- Total contact casts (the gold standard)
- Removable cast boots (examples include DH Walker, Bledsoe Conformer Boot, and Aircast Walker)
- Custom-fabricated ankle-foot orthoses (expensive.)
- Custom and off-the-shelf healing sandals (with Velcro straps, rockers, and a metatarsal bar)
- Half-shoes
- Inlays and insoles (result in minimal pressure reduction in comparison with the options listed above)
- Custom splints (have the longest healing time reported)

8

Complex Wounds

INTRODUCTION

Complex wounds are difficult chronic or acute wounds that defy normal healing and conservative treatment. Common factors of these wounds are conditions such as severe contamination, aggressive infection, cellulitis, extensive tissue necrosis, or crushing injury.

Complex wounds require additional procedures, meticulous surgical debridement, and sophisticated coverage. These wounds are difficult and require a coordinated team from multiple specialties. Working together, thinking outside the proverbial box, being creative, and using innovation help the team achieve the best outcomes for patients with complex wounds. This chapter will cover the assessment and care of necrotizing fasciitis, calciphylaxis, bites, flaps, and grafts.

In this chapter, you will learn:

1. Initial signs and complications that lead to complex wounds.
2. How to recognize necrotizing fasciitis and other wounds with extensive tissue necrosis.
3. Treatment and reconstruction of burn wounds.

INITIAL SIGNS AND COMPLICATIONS OF COMPLEX WOUNDS

Although the wound phase process is the ultimate wound healing model for wounds across the continuum, not all wound hosts are created equally or perfectly. That is a broad statement; therefore, it is important to realize that the host (patient) may be predisposed to complications at any stage (early or late) in the progression of the healing of the wound.

TABLE 8.1   Complications and Symptoms of Complex Wounds

Complication	Type/Example	Signs and Symptoms
Infection	Bacterial Necrotizing fasciitis Viral: Herpes simplex virus (HSV) Yeast: *Candida*	Red streaking, pain, tenderness, warmth, edema. Within 24 to 48 hours: bluish-red dusky surface. Painful, clustered herpetic vesicles. White cottage-cheese-like substance
Autoimmune disorder	Bullous pemphigoid	Itchy patches that lead to firm, strong, and dome-shaped blisters, usually on a limb or in the groin area

Exogenous influences (from outside the body)	Examples: NSAIDs, cytokines, chemotherapeutic agents, psychotropic anticonvulsants, antimicrobial medications, cutaneous radiation injury	Symmetric cutaneous eruptions, uticaria, hemolysis, blisters, and sloughing of skin. Itching, intense reddened area, ulceration
Traumatic complications	Accidental re-injury, self-mutilation or deliberate injury, drug users	Patient pulling dressings off wounds, fragile healed skin. Cutting, cigarette or lighter burns. Puncture sites
Malignancy (neoplasia)	Marjolin's ulcers	Malignant tumor originating from a previous wound (10 to 25 years earlier).
Surgical dehiscence or evisceration	Long-term corticosteroid use, infection, pressure on sutures	Bleeding, redness, swelling, pain, broken sutures, open wound.
Argyria	Silver toxicity	Silver-gray discoloration of skin and nails

TABLE 8.2   Wounds With Extensive Tissue Necrosis

Necrotizing Fascitis (Also Known as Flesh-Eating Bacteria or Streptococcal Gangrene)

Symptoms in first 24 hours	• Usually originates from a minor trauma; initially the wound doesn't appear infected. • Initial regional pain like muscle pain, but it continually gets worse. • Flulike symptoms and intense thirst.
Advanced symptoms within 3 to 4 days	• The painful area begins to swell and a purplish rash appears. • The rash increases in darkness and size, and blackish filled blisters appear. • The wound may have a mottled and necrotic appearance.
Critical symptoms within 4 to 5 days	• The patient experiences toxic shock from the toxins. • Blood pressure drops and the patient becomes unconscious. • Possible other organ failures.
Treatment	• IV antibiotics (single or combination therapy) and IV immunoglobulin. • Aggressive surgical debridement of affected tissue. • Possible hyperbaric oxygen (if the bacteria are anaerobes). • Admit to the burn unit and use silver-impregnated dressings (antimicrobial).

Toxic Epidermal Necrolysis (TEN) (Also Known as Lyell's Disease or Erythema Multiforme)

Symptoms	• Usually originates in adults from a reaction to medication and in children from infection.
	• Fever, flu-like symptoms, and mucous membrane erosions may be the first signs.
	• "With spots" classified as widespread, irregularly shaped erythematous or purpuric blistering macules; very painful.
	• Sheet-like epidermal detachment involves more than 30% of BSA.
	• "Without spots" classified as widespread, large erythematous areas with no discrete lesions; sheet-like epidermal detachment involves more than 10% of BSA.
	• Mucosal surfaces are usually involved.
Treatment	• Discontinue medication, prevent hypothermia, and admit to the burn unit for treatment.

Stevens-Johnson Syndrome (SJS)

Symptoms	• Widespread, irregularly shaped erythematous or purpuric blistering macules.
	• Epidermal detachment involves less than 10% of BSA.
	• Mucosal surfaces are usually involved.
Treatment	• Discontinue medication, prevent hypothermia, and admit to the burn unit for treatment.

BURNS

Know the nearest burn unit, know a resource contact at the burn unit, and know the referral criteria for transferring burn patients. Do not hesitate to use this information. A burn patient's outcome is influenced by early stabilization and resuscitation. Factors affecting the outcome include the depth and size of the burn, the part(s) of the body burned, whether or not smoke inhalation is present, and the patient's age and overall health.

FAST FACTS in a NUTSHELL

Use this indicator to gauge the mortality risk for burn patients:

Percentage of the BSA of the burn + Age of the patient = Mortality risk

Example: A 50-year-old man with a burn of 10% BSA has a 60% mortality risk.

Determining the Severity of a Burn

Depth of a Burn

- First degree (superficial): Red, such as a sunburn.
- Second degree (partial thickness–superficial): Painful blisters and minimal scarring.
- Third degree (partial thickness–deep): Usually dry with ivory coloring at the deepest points; usually requires grafting and produces scarring.
- Fourth degree (full thickness): Skin is destroyed, is white/brown/black in color, and requires removal, grafting, and compression therapy.

Extent of a Burn

Calculate the percentage of the BSA of the burn.

- Rule of 9s

- Lund and Browder Chart
- Rule of Palm (Palm = 1% of BSA)

Type of Burn

- Thermal contact: Scalding, flame, contact, or flash.
- Cold thermal: Frostbite.
- Chemical (acids or bases): Sulfuric acid or hydrofluoric acid.
- Electrical: electric shock, uncontrolled short circuit, or lightning.
- Inhalation: Carbon monoxide poisoning, injury above the glottis, or injury below the glottis.

Referral Criteria

- Second- or third-degree burns of more than 10% of BSA for patients under 10 or over 50.
- Second- or third-degree burns of more than 20% of BSA for all other ages.
- Burns to the face, hands, feet, genitalia, perineum, and major joints.
- Third-degree burns greater than 5% of BSA for any age.
- Circumferential burns.
- Electrical or chemical burns or inhalation.

===================*FAST FACTS in a NUTSHELL*

When in doubt about the severity of a burn and the need for a referral, consult a burn center. To find a list of burn centers nearest you, go to: http://en.wikipedia.org/wiki/List_of_burn_centers_in_the_United_States

SKIN GRAFTS AND TISSUE FLAPS

It is crucial that the wound care nurse act quickly because the patient's skin (being the largest organ of the body)

protects the body from infection, is the sensory contact from injuries, regulates body temperature, and prevents the loss of body fluids.

Essentially, when approaching the appropriate management of large, complex wounds, the wound care nurse should be aware of the prognostic parameters that affect the reconstruction and treatment of the wound. Realistically, this can be considered only through a holistic view of the patient. For instance, the most common treatments for large, complex wounds are skin grafts and tissue flaps. However, smokers have a greater risk of flap failure and are not considered good candidates. Here are the *fast facts* regarding skin grafts and tissue flaps.

TABLE 8.3   Skin Grafts and Tissue Flaps

Skin Grafts: Transplanting healthy skin from one part of a body to a well-vascularized wound area.

Definitions
1. *Allograft: A graft from one person to another (harvested skin from donors).*
2. *Xenograft: A porcine (pig) or bovine (cow) graft.*
3. *Autograft: A graft from one part of the body to another part of the same body.*

Graft Types

Split Thickness (STSG)	• Contains epidermis and superficial dermis and may be meshed. • Grows back from sweat glands and hair follicles, and can cover large areas.
Full Thickness (FTSG)	• Contains epidermis and all of the dermis. • Suitable for covering small defects such as those on the face.

Donor Site	• More painful than the graft; medication is needed before dressing changes.
	• Cleanse, gently pat dry, apply Acticoat, Xeroflo, Mepilex AG, or dry sterile dressings. Some physicians still use Opsite Flexigrid®.

Tissue Flaps: Transplanting healthy skin along with the fat, blood vessels, and possible muscle, and classified by blood supply.

Flap Types

Fasciocutaneous	• Provides padding and superficial coverage.
	• Involves elevation and rotation of the epidermis, dermis, and subcutaneous tissue.
	• May be classified as "random" or "axial" flaps.
Myocutaneous	• Provides good coverage over bony prominences.
	• Involves rotation of all tissue layers (fascia and muscle also).
	• Is well vascularized and contains major vessels.
Sliding Flap	• Is made where the skin is elastic and can be stretched, such as the back of the hand.
Rotation Flap	• Is made by forming the wound into a triangle and rotating the flap into the wound.
	• Is made from sites with good blood supply, such as the scalp, buttocks, thighs, or trunk.
Transposition Flap	• Involves the rotation of a rectangle or square of skin to fill an adjacent wound.

Continued

TABLE 8.3 Skin Grafts and Tissue Flaps *Continued*	
Cultured Skin Graphs and Dermal Substitutes	
Cultured Epithelial Autografts (CEAs)	• Harvesting the patient's own cells to use as a larger epidermal autograft. (Epicel, Laserskin)
Acellular Dermal Allografts	• Composed of cadaveric dermas and used as a scaffold for new tissue to grow through. (AlloDerm, Integra, LifeCell)
Biosynthetic Dressings	
Synthetic Skin Substitutes	• Provide temporary wound coverage. (Biobrane, TransCyte, Dermagraft, Apligraft)

Managing Wounds When a Patient Is Not a Candidate for Graphs or Flaps

Some complex wounds (chronic or acute) are allowed to heal by secondary intention.

Dressing options are dependent upon the wound's size, site, presence or absence of infection, and prognosis. Some common choices are negative-pressure dressings, antimicrobial dressings, Dakin's solution and gauze, and charcoal dressings.

9

Recognizing Atypical Wounds

INTRODUCTION

Atypical wounds can be confusing, even when one has studied the literature and information from wound experts. There is neither universal standardization nor a great deal of evidence-based practice related to such wounds. Hence, when discussing atypical wounds, the wound care nurse looks for an uncommon etiology. These wounds are not common ulcers related to pressure, diabetes, or venous insufficiency. Atypical wounds are in uncommon locations, have unusual or odd appearances, and react indifferently to common treatment therapy. Atypical wounds can progress rapidly into complex wounds (or possibly death) if the underlying cause is not addressed quickly.

In this chapter, you will learn:

1. About atypical wounds, such as those caused by vasculitis, calciphylaxis, and the varicella zoster virus, all of which are difficult, at best, to treat.
2. Some of the most common etiologies of atypical wounds.

117

3. How to understand the type of tissue damage and the patho-physiologic process of viruses.

TYPES OF ATYPICAL WOUNDS AND THEIR ETIOLOGIES

Taking a tissue sample of an atypical wound is perhaps the quickest way to determine the etiology. For instance, vasculitis occurs when the body attacks its own blood vessels. The cause can range from an unknown origin to an infection, an immune system disease, an allergic reaction, a chemical, food, or a malignancy. The symptoms often resemble symptoms of other wound processes, but the treatment prescribed can mean the difference between life and death. A skin biopsy may be the least invasive test to diagnose an etiology.

Vasculitis Disorders

These disorders (called vasculitides) all involve inflammation of the blood vessels, but they differ depending upon which organs with which they are associated. Patients may present with shooting pain in the arms or legs, numbness, and/or asymmetrical weakness in the limbs.

Identifying Skin Features

The skin features of vasculitis disorders include the classic palpable purpura, which are widespread areas of purplish-red spots that may lead to necrosis, ulceration, and possible amputation.

Wound Care Treatment

Initial supportive care of vasculitis patients with mild symptoms of the skin includes limb elevation and compression dressing therapy.

═══════════════════════════════ FAST FACTS in a NUTSHELL

Vasculitis Diseases and Characteristics

Behcet's Disease: Affects the mouth, genitalia, and eyes.

Buerger's Disease: Associated with smokers; affects hands and feet.

Cryoglobulinemia: Recurrent purpura on lower extremities; associated with hepatitis C.

Giant Cell Arteritis: Affects people over 50 years old.

Takayasu's Arteritis: Affects the aorta and vessels leading to the extremities.

Wegener's Granulomatosis: A systemic disease that affects multiple organs.

Calciphylaxis

Calciphylaxis is a metabolic disorder that progresses with vascular calcification. Calciphylaxis is associated with chronic renal failure and is also characterized by necrosis of the skin and fatty tissue. An intact peripheral pulse may differentiate calciphylaxis from other vascular diseases.

Identifying Skin Features

Initially, calciphylaxis is observed as purplish mottling, and then it progresses to bleeding areas that turn into necrotic tissue (dry gangrene). These very painful lesions tend to follow the path of vasculature and are most common on the lower extremities.

Wound Care Treatment

Treatment is dependant upon the severity of calcification and ranges from hyperbaric oxygen to debridement, skin grafting, and/or amputation.

Pyoderma Gangrenosum

Pyoderma gangrenosum is an inflammation process thought to originate from a dysfunctional immune system. There are two types:

- *Typical:* On the legs.
- *Atypical:* On the hands.

Identifying Skin Features

The wound usually appears suddenly as a pustule or blood blister, and often at the site of previous mild trauma. Key features are a violet-purple edge and undermining as the wound rapidly gets larger.

Wound Care Treatment

Treatment is dependent upon the wound, and debridement is usually avoided. Antimicrobial topicals are effective on smaller wounds, but healing is a slow process.

Brown Recluse and Black Widow Spider Bites

Spider bites fall under external causes of atypical wounds. A brown recluse spider bite is usually painless. A black widow's bite causes acute pain, usually within 20 minutes. As the venom is neurotoxic, the patient may experience other side effects such as tremors, muscle cramps, dizziness, and chest pain.

Identifying Skin Features

If brown recluse spider bite symptoms develop, they usually present within 2 to 4 hours after the bite. Fang marks may be present in the center of the site, with a deep-purple plaque around the center, and then a clear halo and redness around the outer edges. This is called "the red, white, and blue sign." Necrotic tissue tends to develop in areas of greater adipose tissue, and there is no antivenin available. The bite of a black widow is called a "target" because it has a pale area surrounded by a red ring. A black widow bite antivenin is available. Severe muscle cramps are a painful development of a black widow bite.

Wound Care Treatment

Brown recluse spider bite treatment options include tetanus immunization (if needed), pain medication, an ice pack (initially), antibiotics if signs of infection are present, Benadryl for itching, and wound care, depending upon wound needs.

Viral Infections That Cause Atypical Wounds

Herpes Simplex (HSV)

HSV-1 (Oral Herpes): Associated with cold sores or fever blisters. It establishes latency in the trigeminal ganglion cells.

Identifying Skin Features: Sores present as uniform, grouped vesicles on a raised base that turn into pustules and weep into a crust, lasting for 2 to 4 weeks.

HSV-2 (Genital and Peri-anal Herpes): Establishes latency in sacral ganglion cells, remains transcriptionally active, reactivates frequently, and may be shed without symptoms or a visible outbreak.

Identifying Skin Features: Lesions present initially as macules and papules, followed by vesicles, pustules, and ulceration, lasting approximately 2 weeks. Lesions may spread from genitalia to perineum and/or buttocks, but they appear as isolated ulcerations rather than rashes.

Two Phases of Infection

- Primary infection: The virus becomes established in a nerve ganglion; this usually occurs in childhood.
- Secondary infection: This usually occurs after sexual contact.

Treatment

- Careful skin care with precautions to avoid spreading the virus.
- Refrigerated antimicrobial hydrogel dressings provide comfort.
- Cleanse with Burrow's solution soaks and keep dry.
- Wash hands after touching infected skin and avoid sunlight.
- Antiviral medications.

Viral infections such as herpes viruses are highly contagious, and once a person is infected, the virus remains in the body for life. For this reason, it is important to recognize the visible sores or wounds. Even though people may become asymptomatic, they can still be contagious to others in a process called viral shedding.

FAST FACTS in a NUTSHELL

Definitions

Asymptomatic: A person is considered asymptomatic if he or she is the carrier of a disease or infection but presently experiences no signs or symptoms.

Viral shedding: The reproduction of host-cell infection as the virus spreads from a cell, or from one part of the body to another, or from the host to another person.

Varicella-Zoster Virus (VZV)

Varicella-zoster virus establishes in a nerve ganglion and causes both chickenpox and herpes zoster virus (shingles). It is transmitted by direct body contact or airborne virus cells.

Chickenpox: Has three stages—raised pink/red papules, then fluid-filled vesicle blisters, and then crusting and scabs.

Treatment

- For the comfort of the patient, keep lights dim, the temperature cool, and the patient out of sunlight.
- Avoidance of aspirin is recommended (related to Reye's syndrome).
- Good hygiene should be maintained, with daily bathing using warm (not hot) water.
- Calamine lotion and zinc oxide barrier are soothing to sores.

Herpes Zoster Virus (Shingles): Presents in the epidermis, with a unilateral vesicular rash along one or two dermatomes. It may be a sign of underlying malignancy.

Symptoms

- Burning, itching, parenthesis, hyeresthesia (oversensitivity), and sharp pains.
- Presents as a rash of vesicular blisters with serous exudate, which become darker as they fill with blood and crust over.

Treatment

- Cleanse with Burrow's solution and apply calamine or topical lidocaine patches.
- Other options are oral steroids, topical capsaicin, or sympathetic blocks.

Many other types of skin damage can lead to atypical wounds. Table 9.1 describes additional atypical wounds.

═══════════════════════*FAST FACTS in a NUTSHELL*

It is acceptable to call a burn center for assistance in the management of patients with large amounts of skin loss. Burn unit staff are knowledgeable and specialized in caring for these patients also.

TABLE 9.1   Atypical Wounds

Wound	Appearance	Treatment
Impetigo (bacterial)	Fluid-filled blisters on a superficial base that form a yellow-tan crust. Satellite lesions from bullous impetigo.	Mupirocin 2%, antimicrobial topical, and good skin hygiene
Cellulitis (inflammation of dermas and subcutaneous tissue)	Red, hot, painful areas, usually where a pre-existing wound is or was.	Antibiotics, debridement if abscessed, and pain medication.
Erysipelas (cellulitis)	Red, hard, swollen area with defined edges that distinguish it from cellulitis. May have red streaks extending outward.	Antibiotics and pain control.
Graft-versus-host disease (GVHD)	Initially, a red skin rash usually affecting the palms and soles of feet that causes itching and darkening skin. Severe cases may result in massive losses of skin.	Immunosuppressants and antiviral medications.
Basal cell carcinomas (cutaneous malignancy)	Varies depending on type: red patch, shiny nodule, thickening skin, or scar tissue.	Excision with biopsy.
Factitial dermatitis (self-inflicted wounds)	Scratches, burns, cuts, bruises, etc., on areas of the body that are easy for the patient to reach.	Psychiatric evaluation and protection of the patient and wound.

Wound Care Treatment and Protocols

10

Understanding Wound Care Guidelines and Protocols

INTRODUCTION

Richard Titmuss defined policy as "the principles that govern action directed towards given ends" and "a consciously chosen course of action (or inaction) directed toward some end."

The medical facility where you work has policies, sometimes called protocols or guidelines. These policies are your baseline of care. Because these guidelines are the common ground for you and your colleagues, it is important to understand the standards (actions and instruction), and purpose (rationale) of a policy or guideline. For instance, hospital policies that relate to patient care are implemented with mission statements, which include standards to provide the highest quality and safest patient care possible, to increase productivity, and to incorporate cost savings.

Any form of policy starts with a knowledge base and insights into the intricacy of the issues at hand. The focus of this chapter will be common guidelines within the specialty of wound care.

In this chapter, you will learn:

1. How wound-care protocols, guidelines, and/or standing orders are developed in medical facilities for standardization.
2. Basic wound care guidelines.

In a perfect clinical world, every facility will have established standardized, evidence-based, skin and wound care guidelines that are adhered to across the continuum of care. However, practically speaking, not all disciplines understand appropriate wound care documentation or the proper use of wound care resources. In an effort to help establish a universal approach, this chapter offers basic wound care guidelines, which may be customized based on the inpatient or outpatient setting.

Exhibit 10.1 shows a policy/procedure template, which is used to develop a policy manual. Exhibit 10.2 shows treatment option guidelines based on best practice.

Exhibit 10.1   Policy/Procedure Template

FACILITY NAME and LOGO   Policy/
Policy/Procedure Manual   Procedure
                                             Number:
                                             Page:
                                             Prepared by:
                                             Date:

Scope: Nursing Personnel

Subject: Wound/Skin Intervention

Purpose: To decrease discrepancies and to provide appropriate and efficient care
Policy: Intervention to prevent skin breakdown, promote optimal wound care, and restore healthy skin
Procedure: Techniques, instructions, and steps

	Effective Date:	Approved by:
Supersedes Policy Dated:	Prepared by:	Approved by:

Exhibit 10.2   Treatment Option Guidelines Based on Best Practice

Conservative Sharp Debridement

Procedure: How often a dressing is changed and specific topical treatment are per physician order.

Preparation

Supplies: Normal saline, gauze, scissors, forceps, scalpel, silver nitrate sticks, dressing.

Pre-medicate the patient, allowing time for medication to take effect.

Don proper attire and prepare the patient (position and dressing removal; measure and photograph wound).

1. Prep the site with antimicrobial cleanser. Cover the area with soaked gauze if necessary, just long enough to help gently remove scabs from healed skin with forceps.
2. Take hold of loose adherent nonviable tissue with forceps, pull tautly, exposing the clear line of dissection. Cut and remove nonviable tissue with scissors. Irrigate the wound.
3. If minor bleeding persists, apply pressure or use silver nitrate.
4. Apply the appropriate dressing depending upon wound size, depth, and drainage.
5. Document the procedure, patient's response, and education of patient/family.

Wounds With Undermining, Tunneling, or Sinus Tract

Procedure: Frequency of dressing changes and specific topical treatment are per physician order.

Continued

Exhibit 10.2 *Continued*

Preparation

Supplies: Normal saline, gauze, primary and secondary dressing choices.

Pre-medicate the patient, allowing time for medication to take effect.

Don proper attire and prepare the patient (position and dressing removal; measure the wound and photograph).

1. Prep the site by irrigating the wound with normal saline or antimicrobial no-rinse cleanser.
2. Fill in tunneling, sinus tract, or undermining by lightly packing one of the following:

Minimal drainage: Hydrogel (antimicrobial or collagen) or impregnated gauze.
Moderate/heavy drainage: Calcium alginate (regular or antimicrobial) or gauze.

3. Be sure to leave a 2-to-4-inch "tail" of packing dressing in the base of the wound for retrieval; if the wound is almost closed, make sure that the 2-to-4-inch tail is outside the opening. Continue to lightly pack the base of the wound, making sure *not* to turn the edges into the wound (causing apiboly).
4. Cover with a secondary dressing (depending upon drainage): Gauze or ABD and stretch-net; other choices: bordered foam, bordered gauze, or silicone.
5. Document the procedure, patient's response, and education of patient/family.

Continued

Exhibit 10.2   *Continued*

Smaller Common Shallow Wounds

Procedure: Frequency of dressing changes and specific topical treatment are per physician order.

Preparation
Supplies: Normal saline, gauze, primary and secondary dressing choices.

Pre-medicate the patient, allowing time for medication to take effect.

Don proper attire and prepare the patient (position and dressing removal; measure the wound and photograph).

1. Prep the site by cleansing the wound with normal saline or antimicrobial no-rinse cleanser.
2. Gently pat dry, and protect periwound skin with no-sting skin prep, lotion, or zinc oxide.
3. Apply the primary dressing:

Minimal drainage: Hydrogel, impregnated gauze, hydrogel sheet, or thin foam.
Moderate drainage: Gauze, alginate, or foam.
Infection present: Silver-based dressing, cadexomer iodine, Bacitracin, or Nystatin.

4. Cover with a secondary dressing (depending upon drainage): Gauze and stretch-net; other choices: bordered foam, bordered gauze, or silicone. The primary and secondary dressing may be the same.
5. Document the procedure, patient's response, and education of patient/family.

Continued

Exhibit 10.2   *Continued*

Smaller Common Deep Wounds (With Craters)

Procedure: Frequency of dressing changes and specific topical treatment are per physician order.

Preparation
Supplies: Normal saline, gauze, primary and secondary dressing choices.

Pre-medicate the patient, allowing time for medication to take effect.

Don proper attire and prepare the patient (position and dressing removal; measure the wound and photograph).

1. Prep the site by irrigating the wound with normal saline or antimicrobial no-rinse cleanser.
2. Gently pat dry; protect periwound skin with no-sting skin prep, lotion, or zinc oxide.
3. Apply the primary dressing:

Minimal drainage: Hydrogel (collagen or antimicrobial), impregnated gauze, TenderWet, or Medihoney.
Moderate/heavy drainage: Medihoney or antimicrobial calcium alginate/collagen/gauze.

4. Cover with a secondary dressing (depending upon drainage): ABD and stretch-net; other choices: bordered foam, bordered gauze, or silicone.
5. Document the procedure, patient's response, and education of patient/family.

Continued

Exhibit 10.2 *Continued*

Massive and Complex Open Wounds

Procedure: Frequency of dressing changes and specific topical treatment are per physician order.

Preparation
Supplies: Normal saline, gauze, primary and secondary dressing choices.

Pre-medicate the patient, allowing time for medication to take effect.

Don proper attire and prepare the patient (position and dressing removal; measure the wound and photograph).

1. Prep the site by irrigating the wound with normal saline or antimicrobial no-rinse cleanser.
2. Gently pat dry; protect periwound skin with no-sting skin prep, lotion, or zinc oxide.
3. Apply the primary dressing option by lining the wound bed with: antimicrobial hydrogel impregnated gauze, silver sulfadiazine 1% cream impregnated gauze, Dakin's solution 0.025% soaked gauze, or acetic acid 0.5% soaked gauze.
4. Lightly pack the wound with fluffed gauze. Apply Montgomery straps or medipore tape.
5. May opt to use negative pressure or suction devices.
6. Document the procedure, patient's response, and education of patient/family.

Continued

Exhibit 10.2 *Continued*

Massive Sloughing of Skin and Burns

Procedure: Frequency of dressing changes and specific topical treatment are per physician order.

Preparation: Do not pop blisters.

Supplies: Normal saline, gauze, scissors, forceps, scalpel, silver nitrate sticks, dressings.

Pre-medicate the patient, allowing time for medication to take effect.

Don proper attire and prepare the patient (dressing removal via bath [shower, tank, or bed bath]), removing dressings and nonviable tissue as you cleanse the patient. Gently dry and remove any further nonviable tissue readily available, and measure and photograph the wounds. Keep the patient warm.

1. For all areas except the face and ears, apply the ordered topical, such as a silver-based topical (gel or silver sulfadiazine), liberally to gauze, spreading evenly if necessary. Cover or spiral wrap areas with saturated gauze.
2. Cover with an appropriate amount of dry sterile dressings. Secure with tape and stretch-net.
3. Apply Ace wraps in a figure 8 over dressings where appropriate.
4. For the face, apply silver-based gel or Bacitracin as needed.
5. For the ears, apply Sulfamylon, dry sterile dressings, and stretch-net.
6. Document the procedure, patient's response, and education of patient/family.

FACILITY NAME and LOGO
PHYSICIAN'S WOUND CARE
ORDER SHEET

Patient Name
Patient FIN #
Date of Birth
Age M/F, Room #
Physician

☐ No Know Allergies ☐ Allergies (list)

☐ Nutrition Consult ☐ Albumin level ☐ Pre-Albumin level ☐ Weight_____

Braden Score: _____ Initiate the following for Braden Scores 16 and lower:
- Pressure reduction mattress
- Pressure relief guidelines for heels & bony prominences (pillows, boots, rail cover)
- Skin integrity guidelines (cleansing, lotion, barrier as needed)
- Eliminate/manage incontinence guidelines (keep patient dry, use air-flow pads)
- Follow turning schedule (implement turn clock)

Preparation for wound treatment:
☐ Cleanse/irrigate wound per guidelines, gently pat dry
☐ Protect peri wound skin with skin protectant per guidelines as needed
☐ Transparent film dressing, change every 3 days and/or PRN
☐ Vaseline/Xeroform gauze, 4x4's, secondary dressing dependent on location.
☐ Iodoform strips, 4x4's, bordered gauze.
☐ Arglaes powder along incision site and bordered gauze.
☐ Do dressing changes on the following days: M T W T F S S (circle)
☐ Notify physician before dressing change
NOTE:

FIGURE 10.1   Physician Wound Care Standing Order Sheet template. The basic guidelines on this sheet may be customized based on the inpatient or outpatient setting.

Continued

Continued

Wound care per Wound Care Consult (consults done within 24 hours)

☐ Notify wound care nurse/department for the following:
- Braden score 16 or lower
- Deep tissue injury or pressure ulcer stage I, II, III, IV
- Vacuum assisted device placement
- Skin tears or new wound injury
- Physician order for wound care consult

Dry eschar on heels/toes:

☐ Paint with betadine, air dry, cover with dry gauze for protection.

Skin tears:

- Category I Apply hydrogel sheet and cotton stretch wrap dressing
- Category II Apply antimicrobial gel and thin foam dressing
- Category III Apply antimicrobial gel and thin foam dressing

Physician Signature: Date: Time:

Orders Noted By: Date: Time:

FIGURE 10.1   Physician Wound Care Standing Order Sheet template. The basic guidelines on this sheet may be customized based on the inpatient or outpatient setting.

═══════════════════════════*FAST FACTS in a NUTSHELL*

Common Topical Options Used in Wound and Burn Care

Ointments: Oil-based, occlusive, lubricating, and effective for approximately 12 hours

- Bacitracin: Gram-positive cocci and bacilli
- Polymyxin B sulfate: Gram-negative organisms
- Neomycin: Broad spectrum

Continued

Continued

- Polysporin: Broad spectrum
- Providone-iodine 10% : Bactericidal spectrum
- Bactroban (Mupirocin): Commonly used in place of sulfa medications

Creams: More water than oil, soothing, and effective for 4 to 12 hours

- Silver sulfadiazine 1%: Antimicrobial, sulfa
- Sulfamylon (Mafenide acetate) 0.5% cream: Antibacterial, sulfa
- Nystatin: Fungicide
- Nitrofurazone 0.2%: Broad antibacterial spectrum
- Gentamicin 0.1%: Gram-negative bacteria

Solutions: Powder form in water, wet-to-moist, and must not be allowed to dry out

- Acetic acid 0.5%: Bactericidal to gram-negative and gram-positive bacteria
- Dakin's solution (sodium hypochlorite) 0.25% to 0.50%: Bactericidal
- Silver nitrate 0.5% solution: Bactericidal, gram-positive bacteria
- Chlorhexinine gluconate 0.5% solution: Antibacterial

Gels: Ionic silver in hydrogel base

- SilvaSorb and Silver-Sept Hydrogels: Antimicrobial

FAST FACTS in a NUTSHELL

The wound and skin guidelines presented in this book may vary depending upon the facility, availability, and rationale. It is important to take into consideration all

Continued

Continued

facets of a patient's wound and skin when choosing treatments. Being competent, understanding rationale, and using good judgment will facilitate the choice of the right treatment and technique.

Skin Care Note Regarding Burns and Massive Skin Sloughing Wounds

Newly epithelialized skin is fragile and may be sensitive for up to a year or more. This is because superficial and partial-thickness burns and wounds heal by regeneration. Remember, epithelial, endothelial, and connective tissue can be reproduced. However, deeper full-thickness wounds heal by scar formation, and structures such as hair follicles, sweat glands, sebaceous glands, subcutaneous tissue, and muscle do not regenerate. Thus, new skin is more likely to be itchy, dry, flaky, and easily sunburned. Education is paramount for the prevention of re-injury. These patients should wear proper attire when out in the sun, such as long sleeves, pants, hats, and sunglasses. Sunscreen is necessary even when it is cloudy. Body and hand soaps should be mild and unscented. Moisturizers should be applied often. A good tip is for patients to keep moisturizer in the bathroom and to use it every time they use the bathroom.

FAST FACTS in a NUTSHELL

Common Soaps and Moisturizers Used for Newly Epithelialized Skin

Consider the choices with which a patient will most likely be compliant. If a patient does not like a greasy feel, no matter how good an ointment is, the patient is not likely to be compliant.

Continued

Continued

Soaps

- Remedy Foaming Body Cleanser
- Remedy Cleansing Body Lotion

Moisturizers

Ointments: Thick and oil-based such as petroleum jelly, contains little water, and are considered occlusive
- Aquaphor ointment

Silicone Blend
- Nutrashield

Creams: Primarily water with emulsified oil
- Remedy Repair Cream
- Eucerin Cream

Lotions: Low viscosity (water-based)
- Lubriderm, Aveeno

Powders: If using an anti-itch powder, choose one that is cornstarch based, not talc.
- Remedy Antifungal Powder (if this is unbearable for the patient, corticosteroid cream may be prescribed.

II

Selecting the Correct Dressings for Optimal Wound Care

INTRODUCTION

Wound care dressings may seem as complex as computer systems, so this chapter is dedicated to helping you make good dressing choices. Even a wound care specialist has to work to stay abreast of manufacturers and the latest technology in wound care offerings. It is a good idea to get to know your wound care representatives. They can offer you brief synopses of their products, and most of them are very respectful of your time. Ask to see a sample, open it and feel it, and compare it with others in the same category.

Starting with the basics, dressings can be divided into two categories: primary and secondary. Primary dressings are those that line the bed of a wound, and secondary dressings are those that secure the primary dressings in place. Sometimes, they are both the same. The wound care nurse needs to be competent in understanding the products by category, their application techniques, and how cost effective they are. Can (and should you) use one product with another? How often do you change a particular dressing? Knowing the answers to these questions is a good example of wound care competency. This chapter will help you become more competent with your wound care choices.

In this chapter, you will learn:

1. The definitions of and indications for advanced wound care and traditional dressings.
2. The advantages and disadvantages of specific advanced wound care and traditional dressings.

WOUND CARE PRODUCTS AND CROSS-REFERENCED DIRECTORIES

The wound care dressings described in the following are classified according to generic category and are cross-referenced by the product name.

TABLE 11.1   Advanced Wound Care Directory

Alginates

Definition: Nonwoven fibers made from processed, sterilized brown seaweed.
Indications: Heavy draining, ulcers, undecompressing, controlled bleeding, crater/cavity, surgical wounds.
Dressing Change Frequency: PRN and/or up to 5 days; document the date and time of the dressing.

Advantages: High absorbency		*Disadvantages:* Require secondary dressing
Primary Dressing	*Primary Dressing*	*Primary Dressing*
+ALGICELL™ by Derma Sciences	+Maxorb™ by Medline	+SILVERCEL™
ALGISITE by Smith & Nephew	MEDIHONEY® by Derma Sciences	+Silverlon® by Argentum
+AQUACEL® by Convatec	+Melgisorb® by Molnlycke	Sorbalgon® by Hartmann
+Arglaes™ powder by Medline	NU-DERM® by Systagenix	Sorbsan® by Mylan Bertek
Curasorb™ by Covidien	+ReliaMed® by ReliaMed	Tegaderm™ high geling by 3M
Kaltostat by ConvaTec	+Restore® by Hollister	Tegaderm™ high integrity by 3M
	+SeaSorb® by Coloplast	

Continued

143

TABLE 11.1 Advanced Wound Care Directory *Continued*

Antimicrobials

Definition: These dressings have an ingredient that is capable of destroying or inhibiting microorganisms.
Indications: Infected wounds or the prevention of infections.

Advantages: Broad-spectrum coverage, controls bioburden   *Disadvantages:* Patient may experience hypersensitivity, require secondary dressing

Primary Dressing	Agent Used in Primary Dressing	Dressing Change Frequency
+Di-Dak-Sol® by Century	Dakins solution 0.0125%	Compare product package insert with the secondary dressing package insert. The product insert that requires re-application more often is the proper one to go by. Use good judgment.
+Iodoflex by Smith & Nephew	Cadexomer Iodine	
+Hydrofera Blue by Healthpoint	Gentian Violet/Methylene Blue	
+Tegaderm Ag Mesh by 3M	Silver	
+XCell® by Medline	Cellulose and PHMB	

Burn and Contact Layer Dressings

Definition and Indications: These dressings offer antimicrobial activity and sizes that are practical for large burns and traumatic wounds. The contact layer dressing protects the wound base while allowing fluid to pass through to the secondary dressing.

Advantages: Wound drainage is wicked to the secondary dressing, protects wound base

Disadvantages: Patient may experience hypersensitivity, require secondary dressing

Primary Burn Dressings	Contact Layer Dressings	Dressing Change Frequency
+Acticoat by Smith & Nephew Intersorb® by Covidien +SelectSilver® by Milliken +Silverlon® by Argentum	ADAPTIC® by Systagenix DERMANET® by DeRoyal N-TERFACE® by Winfield Mepitel® by Molnlycke Oil-Emulsion by Medline Petrolatum Gauze by Medline Restore® Contact layer by Hollister Silon-TSR® by BMS Telfa™ Clear by Covidien Tegaderm™ Contact layer by 3M Xeroflo® by Covidien	Surgical dressings: Initial application may be performed in surgery and have specific orders with them. Always check orders for timing of surgical takedown and reapplication.

Collagen Dressings

Definition: Collagen, usually bovine, porcine, or equine derived; aid fibroblast production; contribute to new tissue growth.

Indications: Ulcers, donor sites, partial-/full-thickness wounds, grafts, surgical wounds

Continued

TABLE 11.1 Advanced Wound Care Directory *Continued*

Advantages: May be used with antimicrobials, available in different forms

Disadvantages: Not acceptable for necrotic wounds, require secondary dressing

Primary	Derived From:	Dressing Change Frequency
Biopad® sponge by SkinSafe	Equine	Compare collagen product package insert with the secondary dressing package insert. Collagen inserts range in reapplication of dressing from twice a day in heavily draining wounds to whenever the secondary dressing is changed. Use good judgment.
+BIOSTEP by Smith & Nephew	Porcine	
CellerateRX® by WCI	Type 1 (1/100 size) collagen	
CollaSorb® by Hartmann	Bovine	
FIBRACOL™ by Systagenix	Combined with alginate	
Medifil® particles by BioCore	Bovine	
+PROMOGRAM® PRISMA™	Matrix cellulose	
+Puracol™ by Medline	Bovine type1	
+SilvaKollagen® Gel by DermaRite	Hydrolystate of collagen	
Stimulen™ Powder by Southwest	Modified	

Compression and Unna Boots

Definition: Dressings that compress the area, help circulation and blood flow back to the heart, and reduce edema.

Indications: Venous ulcers, control of scar hypertrophy (in burns).

Dressing Change Frequency: Burn patients require 23-hour/day compression; Unna boots and other compression modes are used up to a week. Check product insert/order/guidelines.

Advantages: Length of dressing changes (up to a week), cost

Disadvantages: Cannot be used with arterial disease; proper application takes training and practice.

Compression	Elastic Wraps and Unna Boots	Stockings
2-Layer: 18–25 mmHg Pressure	*1-Layer and Elastic Wraps*	*Stockings*
Coban™ 2 Layer by 3M	CoFlex-LF2 by Andover	Stocking system by Carolon
3-Layer: 30–40 mmHg Pressure	Setopress® by Molnlycke	
DYNA-FLEX™ by Systagenix	SurePress® by ConvaTec	
PROFORE LITE by Smith & Nephew	*Unna Boot*	
PROGUIDE by Smith & Nephew	Econo-Paste® by Hartmann	
ThreeFlex™ by Medline	Gelocast® by BSN	
ThreePress® by Hartman	Primer® by Derma Science	
4-Layer: 30–40 mmHg Pressure	Unna-Flex® by ConvaTec	
ThreeFlex™ by Medline	VISCOPASTE by Smith & Nephew	
FourPress® by Hartman		
PROFORE by Smith & Nephew		

Sequential Intermittent Compression Systems: Talley Medical or Thermo Tek

Continued

147

TABLE 11.1   Advanced Wound Care Directory   *Continued*

Debriders: Enzymatic, Polyacrylate, Devices

Definition: Devices that loosen and dissolve nonviable tissue
Indications: Wounds with eschar, necrosis, or slough

Advantages: Reduce bioburden, alternative for patients who are not candidates for sharp surgical debridement		*Disadvantages:* May damage or macerate skin surrounding nonviable tissue, cannot be used with antimicrobial metals, high cost

Debriders	*Debriders*	*Dressing Change Frequency*
Collagenase Santyl® by HealthPoint Cadexomer Iodine Iodosorb by Smith & Nephew *Devices: Ultrasonic* Qoustic System™ by Arobella Sonoca® 180 by Soring	*Polyacrylate* TenderWet™ by Medline *Maggots* Creature Comforts™ by Monarch *Devices: High-Pressure Steam* Versajet by Smith & Nephew	Compare the debrider package insert with the physician's order. Debriders differ in range as to reapplying. Use good judgment.

Foams

Definition: Highly absorptive polyurethane dressing that wicks exudate away from wound.
Indications: Appropriate for any wound, matching foam (thick or thin) to drainage amount.
Dressing Change Frequency: PRN and/or up to 5 days; document the date and time of dressing. Check the product insert.

Advantages: Variety of sizes, shapes, and types; ease of application and removal	*Disadvantages*: May macerate skin surrounding skin if not changed appropriately cannot be used on dry eschar.

Foams

Foams	
+ALLEVYN by Smith & Nephew	Restore® (with TRIACT Technology) by Hollister
+Biatain® (foam/hydrocolloid base) by Coloplast	SorbaCell® (large foam filler) by Derma Sciences
	Tegaderm™ by 3M
CoFlex® (foam/cohesive bandage) by Andover	Tielle® (hydropolymer) by Systagenix
Lyfoam® (fenestrated version) by Molnlycke	Versiva® XC (gelling Foam) by ConvaTec
+Mepilex® (silicone technology) by Molnlycke	XTRASORB® (polymer based foam) by Derma Sciences
+Optifoam™ (high MVTR) by Medline	
PermaFoam® (high MVTR) by Hartmann	
+PolyMem® by Ferris	

Continued

TABLE 11.1 Advanced Wound Care Directory *Continued*

Genetically Engineered Growth Factors, Extracellular Matrix, and Skin Substitutes

Definitions: Extracellular matrix is created from porcine small intestines, skin substitutes are processed from human tissue (living cells), and genetically engineered growth factors are formulated into gels.

Indications: Wounds with poor circulation (arterial), graft sites, and chronic slowly healing or nonhealing wounds.

Dressing Change Frequency: These dressings are bioabsorbable. Perform dressing changes per order.

Advantages: Enhance the body's healing capability   *Disadvantages:* High cost, may need to be refrigerated

Genetically Engineered Growth Factors	Extracellular Matrix	Skin Substitutes
AutoloGel System™ by Cytomedix	MatriStem™ by Medline	AlloDerm® by LifeCell
Regranex® by Systagenix	Oasis® Matrix by Healthpoint	Apligraf® by Organogenesis
		Dermagraft® by Advanced BioHealing
		Integra™ by Integra LifeScience
		Biobrane® by Smith & Nephew

Hydrocolloids

Definition: Wafer dressings usually derived from pectin or gelatin. Hydrocolloids are occlusive and are the most adhesive dressings available. Reacting with the wound bed, they turn into a gelatinous covering.
Indications: Primary/secondary dressing for minimally draining wounds. Preventive dressing on nonfragile skin.

Advantages: Occlusive, autolytic debridement, variety of sizes, shapes, and forms	Disadvantages: Not recommended for heavily draining wounds, are difficult to remove, emit odor with removal	
Hydrocolloids	*Hydrocolloids*	*Dressing Change Frequency*
+Comfeel® by Coloplast	NU-DERM® by Systagenix	Compare the product package insert with the physician's order. These usually have up to 3-, 5-, or 7-day reapplication times. Use good judgment.
DuoDerm® by ConvaTec	REPLICARE by Smith & Nephew	
Exuderm OdorShield™ by Medline	Restore® by Hollister	
	Tegaderm™ by 3M	
FlexiCol® by Hartmann	TIELLE by Systagenix	
Hydrocol® by Mylan Bertek	Ultec® by Covidien	
Medihoney™ by Derma Science		

Continued

TABLE 11.1   Advanced Wound Care Directory   *Continued*

Hydrogel Dressings

Definition: Usually water or glycerin-based in the form of gels, sheets, or impregnated in gauze.
Indications: Painful wounds, burns, skin tears, dry wounds, partial- and full-thickness wounds.
Dressing Change Frequency: Check the product insert; varies from 1, 3, or 5 days, depending upon delivery system.

Advantages: Flexibility in wound, soothing, variety of forms and sizes

Disadvantage: May require secondary dressing, not recommended for heavily draining wounds

Hydrogel Gel	Hydrogel Sheets	Impregnated Hydrogel Gauze
+AmeriGel® by Amerx	AquaClear® sheet by Hartman	AmeriGel® by Amerx
CURAFIL® by Covidien	Aquaflo disk by Covidien	CURAGEL® by Covidien
CURASOL® by Healthpoint	AquaSite® by Derma Sciences	Dermagran by Derma Sciences
Dermagran® by Derma Sciences	CURACEL® Island by Covidien	Elta® by Swiss-American
DuoDERM Gel by ConvaTec	CURACEL® sheet by Covidien	+ReliaMed® hydrogel by ReliaMed
Elta® Gel by Swiss-American	Derma-Gel™ sheet by Medline	Restore® by Hollister
Hypergel® by Molnlycke	Elasto-Gel™ by Southwest	SkinTegrity® by Medline
INTRASITE Gel by Smith & Nephew	FLEXIGEL sheet by Smith & Nephew	
Normlgel® by Molnlycke	NU-GEL® by Systagenix	
Purilon® Gel by Coloplast		

RadiaCare™ Gel by Carrington
Restore® by Hollister
SAF-Gel® by ConvaTec
+SilvaSorb® Gel Medline
+Silver Sept™ by Anacapa
SkinTegrity® Gel by Medline
SOLOSITE Gel by Smith & Nephew
Wound-Be-Gone® by Wake
WounDres® by Coloplast

RadiaDres™ by Carrington
SilvaSorb® sheets by Medline
Skintegrity® sheet by Medline
Toe-Aid™ by Southwest

Odor-Absorbing Dressings

Definition: These dressings contain activated charcoal to absorb odors.
Indications: Malodorous, partial- and full-thickness wounds, fungating wounds.
Dressing Change Frequency: Check the product insert and compare it with the secondary dressing insert.

Advantages: Can be used as a primary or secondary dressing, helps neutralize offensive odors

Disadvantages: High cost, may require a secondary dressing

Dressings

+ACTISORB® Systagenix
Restore® foam/fabric by Hollister

CarboFlex by ConvaTec

LYOFOAM® C foam by Molnlycke

Continued

TABLE 11.1   Advanced Wound Care Directory   *Continued*

Scar Therapy Dressings

Definition: These dressings may help reduce the appearance of scars. This is not a usual wound care product category; however, it is helpful to have knowledge of them for patients or colleagues when they ask.

Advantages: These products may reduce hypertrophic or keloid scars from developing

Disadvantages: Not all scars respond to scar therapy, especially keloids (incorporate this information into discharge teaching)

Development Control	Color Correction	Tip
Mepiform® by Molnlycke Oleeva Clear® by BMS CICA-CARE by Smith & Nephew	Exuviance® by Neo Strata Mederma® by Mederma Remedy™ by Medline	Maintain good pain management (itching) Maintain good nutrition Maintain good hygiene

Transparent Films

Definition: Clear film dressings made from polyurethane. Added polymers allow gas and moisture vapor to escape.
Indications: Minimally draining wounds with nonfragile surrounding skin. Not for use on patients with tape allergies.
Dressing Change Frequency: Check the product insert; up to 7 days and as needed.

Advantages: Fewer dressing changes; reduce friction; variety of sizes, shapes, and forms; is transparent

Disadvantages: Adherence to fragile skin, possible maceration, cause tape burns if not properly removed

Films	Correct Removal of Films
+Arglaes™ by Medline BIOCLUSIVE® by Systagenix Blisterfilm® by Covidien Comfeel® by Coloplast Elta® by Swiss-American Hydrofilm® by Hartmann	Mepore® by Molnlycke OPSITE® by Smith & Nephew ReliaMed® by ReliaMed Suresite® by Medline +Tegaderm™ by 3M	Take hold of the edge of film with one hand, stabilizing it in place with the other hand. Gently stretch horizontally and close to the skin. Walk your fingertips across the dressing slowly, stretching it as you go. This is a slow process, but it minimizes pain.

Note: A + indicates whether the product is/or offers an antimicrobial version; hence, these products will be under their generic category – not under the antimicrobial category.

TABLE 11.2   Traditional Wound Care Directory

Gauze Dressings

Definition: Woven or nonwoven, adherent or nonadherent, sterile or unsterile roll, pad, and sponge dressings made in a variety of sizes and shapes.

Indications: Not all gauze dressings are the same. Check the package insert to compare with the desired effects.

Dressing Change Frequency: Compare the product insert with the dressing change order.

Advantages: Available in a variety of sizes, shapes, and forms; moist wound environment, protection, mechanical debrider

Disadvantages: May adhere to fragile skin, possible maceration, may dry out

Absorptive	Primary and Packing	Secondary and Wrapping
ABD Pads by Medline	+CURITY® packing strips by Covidien	CONFORM® stretch by Covidien
Abdominal Pads by ReliaMed	+Excilon® by Covidien	Cover-Roll® by BSN
Cosmopore® by Hartmann	KERLIX® packing strips by Covidien	COVRSITE by Smith & Nephew
Drawtex Capillary by Drawtex	Packing strips by Medline	Duform® stretch by Derma Sciences
EXU-DRY by Smith & Nephew	Sorbalux® sponge by Hartmann	KERLIX® Rolls by Covidien
XTRASORB™ by DermaScience	+TELFA® pad by Covidien	TELFA® Island by Covidien
	TheraGauze™ by Soluble Systems	

Dressing Retention

Definition: Elastic and tubular stretch dressings, cut to size and shape, hold dressings in place while allowing ease of movement and air circulation.

Indications: For patients with tape allergies, difficult areas to dress (because of gravity or friction), or restlessness.

Dressing Change Frequency: Per order for primary dressing and as needed.

Advantages: May be lifted for assessment of wounds and put back in place, very inexpensive, no tape burns		*Disadvantages*: Application learning curve for using the right size

Stretch-Net	*Stretch Cotton Wrap*	*Garments*
Elastic Net by Medline Flexinet® by Derma Science Surgilast® by Derma Science	Medigrip by Medline Tubigrip™ by Molnlycke	Arm Sleeve by Medline Glen-Sleeve® by Derma Sciences Heel and Elbow Protectors by ReliaMed Tubifast™ by Molnlycke

Miscellaneous

Definition: Wound care products that additionally support a wound, patient, and nurse.

Advantages: Enhance nursing care and wound care outcomes	*Disadvantages*: High cost, contract, availability

Continued

TABLE 11.2   Traditional Wound Care Directory   *Continued*

Prepping Products	*Dressing Take-Downs*	*Assessment*
Adhesive Remover Wipes by ReliaMed Alcohol Preps by Covidien Foam-Tipped Applicators by Puritan Povidone/Iodine Solution by Medline	CarraScent™ by Carrington Sani-Zone™ by Anacapa Suture Removal Tray by Medline	ARANZ Silhouette by Aranz Dopplers by Briggs or Summit Interface Pressure Monitor by Talley PPRS photo system by Briggs

Wound Cleansers

Definition: Cleansers made specifically for wounds have a pressure of between 4 and 15 psi. Bottle sizes vary, ingredients vary from normal saline to antimicrobial, surfactants, and/or preservatives. Check labels.
Indications: For cleansing or irrigating all types of wounds.

Advantages: A variety of delivery methods (spray or stream), no-rinse, noncytotoxic	*Disadvantages:* Some solutions may be toxic to cells, improper spray distance can affects psi

Saline-Based Cleansers	*Antimicrobial and/or Antiseptic Cleansers*	*Scrub (Friction) Cleansers*
Amerigel® by Amerx Dermal by Smith & Nephew Restore® by Restore	+Anasept™ by Anacapa +MicroKlenz™ by Medline	Optipore® sponge by ConvaTec

158

SAF-Clens® by ConvaTec
Sea-Clens® by Coloplast
Skintegrity® by Medline

Ultradex™ E-Z scrub sponge by BD
[3% chloroxylenol (PCMX), and
emollients]

Wound Closures

Definition: These products help bring the edges of a wound together. Tapes hold dressings in place.
Indications: For gaping complex wounds and wounds left open to heal by tertiary intention.

Advantages: Variety of sizes, shapes, and forms

Disadvantages: Adherence to fragile skin,
application learning curve, cause tape burns if not
properly removed

Dressings	Devices/Expanders	Skin Adhesive and Tape
Adhesive Surgical Dressing by Medline	S.T.A.R. device by WoundTek	Dermabond® by Ethicon
DP® Direct Pressure by DP	DermaClose RC by Woundcare	Mefix® by Molnlycke
Medi-Strips® by Medline		Megazine Pink™ by Medline
Montgomery Straps by Medline		Variety of Tapes by Medline
Steri-Strip™ by 3M		Variety of Tapes by 3M

Exhibit II.I   Skin and Wound Care Guidelines

Reddened Area Stage I

Stage I: An area where the epidermis is intact & the erythema (reddened skin) does not resolve within 30 minutes of pressure relief.
OVER A BONY PROMINENCE
MANAGEMENT
*Reposition EVERY 2 hrs. & PRN
*Relief by pillows
*Off-loading-heel-lift boots
TREATMENT
Skin protectant, or barrier ointment, or foam dressing for protection
IX for Moisture:
Cleanse after each incontinence episode with cleanser or wipes. Apply skin protectant PRN.

Reddened/Denuded Buttocks

Only stage if over bony prominence or caused by pressure.
Excoriated, Friction, Shear areas: Likely due to exposure to urine and stool.
MANAGEMENT
USE underpads that wick moisture away from patient skin.
TREATMENT
Apply zinc barrier after peri-care & PRN until improved; then resume skin protectant for prevention.
Persistent redness/satellite lesions:
Consider need for antifungal powder.

Skin Tear

Do **not** stage; traumatic wound not pressure related.
Category I
A skin tear without tissue loss.
Category II
A skin tear with partial tissue flop loss.
Category III
A skin tear with complete tissue flap loss.

Continued

Exhibit 11.1 *Continued*

MANAGEMENT
Coverbed railings with padding. Use skin protectant & tubular stockingette on arms &/or legs for protection.
TREATMENT Cleanse wound. Approximate wound edges if needed & apply barrier ointment
DRESSINGS
thin or regular foam, or hydrogel sheet
PREVENTION antimicrobial gel, foam dressings, or powder

Deep Tissue Injury

Purple or maroon localized area of discoloured intact skin or blood-filled blister due to damage of underlying soft tissue from pressure &/or shear.
MANAGEMENT
Reposition EVERY 2 hrs. & PRN Relief by pillows Off-loading, heel-lift boots, foam cushions
TREATMENT Cleanse & dry area.
Blister Intact: Protect with skin protectant lotion, & observe frequently to keep further injury from occurring.
Blister Broken: Antimicrobial gel. Cover with foam. Assess daily, change per facility/product guidelines & PRN.

Partial Thickness Stage II

A Stage II bridges over from a Stage I as a blister (fluid pocket denotes epidermis lifts from dermis). Following, an area of partial thickness loss of skin layers involving the epidermis & possibly penetrating into but not through the dermis.
MANAGEMENT
Reposition every 2 hrs. & PRN Relief by pillows Off-loading, heel-lift boots, foam cushions
TREATMENT Intact Blister Apply skin protectant. **Abrasion, Shallow Crater, Partial Thickness**
Non-minimal draining: Antimicrobial gel & foam dressing.
Draining: antimicrobial alginate & gauze or foam. Assess daily, change per facility/product guidelines & PRN.
*Consult wound team if no improvement.

Continued

Exhibit 11.1 *Continued*

Full Thickness Stage III

Full thickness skin loss involving damage or necrosis of subcutaneous tissue, which may extend down to but not through the
underlying fascia. The ulcer presents clinically as a deep creater
with or without undermining of adjacent tissue.

Full Thickness Depth Stage III

Full thickness skin loss with extensive tissue destruction, necro-
sis or damage to muscle, bone, or supporting structures (tendon,
joint capsule, etc.).
MANAGEMENT
Reposition EVERY 2 hrs. & PRN Relief by pillows Off-loading,
heel-lift boots, foam cushions
TREATMENT
Gently cleanse wound. Apply sting-free liquid barrier to sur-
rounding tissue and let dry.
Non-minimal draining:
Granulating, Clean Wound Beds:
Gently place antimicrobial impregnated gel gauze into wound
base. Cover with foam or gauze/elastic net. Assess daily, change
per facility/product guidelines & PRN.
Moderate to Heavy Drainage Minimal Non-Viable Tissue
Apply Alginate, boister with 4X4s. Use foam or ABD/elastic net
for secondary dressing. Assess daily, change per facility/product
guidelines & PRN.
Tunneled Wounds with small openings: Use antimicrobial powder on lightly moistened packing strips. Gently place into tunneled areas making sure to leave tail in base of wound. Use foam
or ABD elastic net for secondary dressing. Assess daily, change
per facility/product guidelines & PRN.
KEEP TENDONS MOIST IF VISIBLE.

Full Thickness Slough

Unable to stage.
Moist devitalized stringy fibrinous tissue that appears yellowy,
white ot gray in appearance.

Continued

Exhibit 11.1   *Continued*

Full Thickness Eschar

Unable to stage.
Firm, dry, leathery, black, dead tissue.
MANAGEMENT
Reposition EVERY 2 hrs. & PRN Relief by pillows Off-loading, heel-lift boots, foam cushions
NECROTIC WOUND TREATMENT
Gently cleanse wound. Apply sting-free liquid barrier to surrounding tissue and let dry.
DRY HEEL ESCHAR
Leave open to air or protect with dry gauze.
NEVER ATTEMPT TO DEBRIDE INTACT ESCHAR ON HEELS
If breaks open:
Apply betadine, protect with dry gauze, assess for surgical consult.
SLOUGH &/OR ESCHAR OPTIONS
Minimal amount: polyacrylate pads or encymatic debridement. Use foam or gauze/ elastic net for secondary dressing. Assess daily, change per facility/product guidelines & PRN.
Moderate to heavy amount: Alginate or Dakins Solution & surgical consult. Bolster with gauze/elastic net for secondary dressing. Assess daily, change per facility/product guidelines & PRN.
KEEP TENDONS MOIST IF VISIBLE.

═══════════════*FAST FACTS in a NUTSHELL*

Dressing Applications and Reapplications

Dressing Applications: Patients and wounds are either digressing, unchanging, or progressing. Be prepared. Choose the primary dressing based on whether the wound is dirty or clean, wet or dry, and deep or shallow. Choose the secondary dressing based on minimal or heavy drainage and the condition of surrounding skin.

Continued

Continued

Reapplication of Dressings: Dressing reapplications are based on physician's orders, product inserts, and facility guidelines. Compare these and use good judgment. For example, if the primary dressing's product insert indicates reapplication twice a day and you choose a secondary dressing whose product insert indicates reapplication up to 7 days, you will be changing the dressings according to the shortest reapplication time. Make sure that your dressing selections are safe, appropriate, and cost effective.

12

Using Adjunctive Therapies

INTRODUCTION

Adjunctive therapies are treatment modalities that enhance primary wound care treatment. The wound care nurse may or may not initiate adjunctive therapy; however, it is imperative to understand these modalities, their indications, contraindications, advantages, disadvantages, and trade names.

In this chapter, you will learn:

1. The definitions of and indications for different wound care adjunctive therapies, such as negative pressure, electrical stimulation, hyperbaric oxygenation, pulsed lavage, and lymphatic drainage therapy.
2. The advantages and disadvantages of specific wound care adjunctive therapies.

ADJUNCTIVE THERAPIES AND DIRECTORIES

The specific therapies described in the following are classified according to generic category and cross referenced by the product name. Following the guidelines and/or protocols for these modalities is crucial. These treatment modalities may be highly efficient or highly detrimental, depending upon the provider's technique, knowledge, and/or application. There is limited evidence regarding efficacy and effectiveness with adjunctive therapies. However, nurses certified within these specialties, and technicians and physical therapists working with these modalities can offer a wealth of knowledge based on hands-on experience.

═══════════════════════════════*FAST FACTS in a NUTSHELL*

Electrical Stimulation Terms

- *Alternating current:* Biphasic, the direction of current constantly switches direction, back and forth.
- *Current of injury:* The current that flows through wound fluid when tissue is damaged. This current disappears when tissue heals and becomes dry. This is the evidence behind moist wound healing.
- *Frequency:* The number of pulse cycles per second.
- *Galvanotaxis:* The directional movement of cells in relation to a current.
- *Polarity:* Every electrical circuit has a negative and positive pole. The current flows from one to the other.
- *Pulse duration:* The interval of time when the current is flowing.
- *Voltage:* The force that drives an electric current. (Voltage = Current × Resistance)
  - ○ Low-voltage devices: 60–100 V
  - ○ High-voltage devices: 100–500 V

Exhibit 12.1   Electrical Stimulation

Electrical Stimulation (HCPCS Code E0769)

Definition: Transferring electrical current to a wound; based on studies related to a healthy body retaining electrical current. The electrical current is applied to the wound bed and surrounding skin via electrodes and waveforms.

Indications: Recalcitrant arterial, diabetic, or venous ulcers, and chronic Stage III and Stage IV pressure ulcers

Advantages: Decreases pain, increases oxygen perfusion, can be used on infected wounds	*Disadvantages:* Length of treatment, consistency, reimbursement (unattended or attended coding)

Four types of electrical stimulation have been applied to wound care:

- Low-voltage, continuous micro-amperage direct current: It has a continuous, monophasic waveform, and the voltage does not vary with time.
- High-voltage pulsed current (HVPC): It has a waveform of paired short-duration pulses with a long interpulse interval. (This method is most common.)
- Low-voltage pulsed microamperage current: It has an interrupted direct current, a wide rectangular pulse width, and a short interpulse interval.
- Low-voltage pulsed milliamperage current: It has symmetric biphasic pulses and is commonly known as TENS (transcutaneous electrical nerve stimulator).

Continued

Exhibit 12.1 *Continued*

Treatment Protocol

- Gather supplies, premedicate the patient for pain and position the patient, remove the dressing, and cleanse the wound, making sure no petrolatum products remain in the wound.
- Line the wound bed with normal saline-soaked or hydrogel-impregnated gauze.
- Place the electrode over the wet gauze and cover (lightly pack) with dry gauze. Secure the dressing.
- Attach aluminum foil with an alligator clip to the stimulator lead.
- Next, place the dispersive electrode proximally to the wound (if possible), and place a damp washcloth under this electrode. Make sure that the electrode is not overlapping the edge of the washcloth, and secure it for good contact with the skin.

Wounds in Inflammation Phase: Stimulator Settings

- Polarity: Negative
- Pulse rate: 100 to 128 pulse per second (pps)
- Intensity: 100 to 150 volts
- Duration: 60 minutes
- Frequency: 5 to 7 times a week, once daily

Wounds in Epithelialization Phase: Stimulator Settings

- Polarity: Alternate 3 days negative followed by 3 days positive
- Pulse rate: 64 pps
- Intensity: 100 to 150 volts

Continued

Exhibit 12.1 *Continued*

- Duration: 60 minutes
- Frequency: 6 times a week, once daily

Post-Treatment

- Gently remove electrodes and apply a dressing per order and wound requirements.

Side Effects: Pain, irritation under electrode placement.

Contraindications: Placing electrodes close to the heart; patients with osteomyelitis, a pacemaker, or a malignancy.

Product Name: FREMS™ (Frequency Rhythmic Electrical Modulation System) by Lorenz NeuroVasc®

Tip: To deliver pulsed electrical stimulation, these parameters must be set: amperage, duration of pulse, frequency, length of interpulse interval, placement of cathode and anode, and pulse width.

Exhibit 12.2 Hyperbaric Oxygenation

Hyperbaric Oxygenation Therapy (HCPCS Code C1300)

Definition: Hyperbaric oxygenation therapy (HBOT) is the breathing of 100% oxygen in a monochamber or multiperson hyperbaric chamber, which delivers pressures of 2.0 to 2.4 times the normal atmospheric pressure (ATA). The treatment dissolves oxygen into the plasma, increases oxygen tension in hypoxic areas, reduces edema, and enhances white blood cell activity at the wound site.

Continued

Exhibit 12.2 *Continued*

Indications: Crush injuries, necrotizing fascitis, chronic refractory osteomyelitis, thermal burns, compromised skin grafts, and epidermal flaps (not all inclusive).

Advantages:	*Disadvantages:* No
Vasoconstriction,	direct patient contact,
increased oxygenation	cosmetic products must be
of tissue	removed, difficult to monitor

Patient Education to Prevent Complications

- Teach air-equalization techniques to prevent "ear squeeze."
- Remind the patient not to hold his or her breath, related to possible pneumothorax.
- Instruct the patient to remove personal items and cosmetics, such as contact lenses, perfume, hairspray, and lip balm.
- Remove dressings from the wound, especially petrolatum dressings.
- Assess for medication changes, diabetic control, and anxiety.

Treatment Protocol

Treatments vary but usually consist of 2-hour sessions, several times a week, on an outpatient basis.

- To be covered by Medicare, a physician must be present during the entire treatment.
- UHMS protocols and physician preferences are considered standard guidelines.

Side Effects: Claustrophobia, aural barotraumas (ear squeeze), myopia, tension pneumothorax

Continued

Exhibit 12.2   *Continued*

Contraindications: Patients receiving bleomycin, cis-platinum, Sulfamylon, and disulfiram, and patients with untreated pneumothorax, pregnancy, a known malignancy, emphysema, bronchitis, or hyperthermia.

Product Names: Perry Baromedical Hyperbaric Therapy Systems, Sechrist Industries Monoplace Hyperbaric Chambers

Hyperbaric oxygenation is an adjunctive therapy that is expensive, time consuming, and of no benefit when used inappropriately. Hence, this treatment has been under much scrutiny. Patient selection should include a thorough assessment and the hypoxic state of the wound.

================*FAST FACTS in a NUTSHELL*

Gas Laws on Which Hyperbaric Oxygenation Is Based

Boyle's Law: The absolute pressure and volume of a gas are inversely proportional when kept at a constant temperature.

Charles's Law: Gases and vapors expand when heated.

Henry's Law: The solubility of a gas in a liquid, at a certain temperature, is proportional to the pressure of the gas above the liquid.

Hyperbaric nursing requires certification and may be obtained through the Baromedical Nurses Association (BNA) at http://www.hyperbaricnurses.org.

For more information visit the Undersea & Hyperbaric Medical Society at http://www.uhms.org

================================= *FAST FACTS in a NUTSHELL*

Lymphatic Drainage Therapy Procedure Terms

- *Proximal clearing:* To prevent overloading the chest and trunk, manual lymphatic drainage starts proximally, clearing the chest and trunk first. Then the affected limb is treated.
- *Light pressure:* To prevent damage to lymph capillaries, light, gentle pressure is applied for absorption.
- *Dynamic pressure:* A work-and-release action by calibrated-system inflation and immediate-deflation timed cycles.
- *Timing:* A succession of individual chambers deliver 1- to 3-second applications of pressure.
- *Skin stretch:* A special stretch fabric that delivers stretch against the skin to manipulate lymph capillaries.
- *Directional pressure:* Distal-to-proximal directional pressure to redirect fluid away from swollen areas.
- *Repetition:* Repetitive work-and-release in each region.

Exhibit 12.3 Lymphatic Drainage Therapy

Lymphatic Drainage Therapy (HCPCS Code E0652)

Definition: A segmented pneumatic compression device with calibrated inflation/deflation through 27 to 32 chambers, built into adjustable stretch fabric. The system redirects lymph fluid to other regions of the body.

Indications: Primary lymphedema patients, patients with lymphedema secondary to cancer, surgery, venous insufficiency, trauma, infection, post-mastectomy edema, and stasis dermatitis (not all inclusive).

Continued

Exhibit 12.3 *Continued*

Advantages: Uses physiological principles of manual lymphatic drainage (MLD) therapy without the manual labor of MLD

Disadvantages: Eligibility for reimbursement, keeping a consistent schedule

Note: For more information on lymphedema, go online to The National Lymphedema Network at http://www.lymphnet.org.

Treatment Protocol

Complete decongestive therapy (CDT) includes:

- Flexitouch® used as adjunctive therapy for MLD.
- Meticulous skin and nail care.
- Compression bandaging.
- Decongestive exercise (water exercises).
- Instruction in self-management (elevation of the affected limb, being compliant with compression).

Side Effects: Breathing issues with pleural effusions

Contraindications: Pulmonary edema, thrombophlebitis, congestive heart failure, deep vein thrombosis

Product Name: Flexitouch®

Exhibit 12.4   Negative-Pressure Wound Therapy

Negative-Pressure Therapy (HCPCS Code E2402; Supplies A6550, A7000)

Definition: Negative-pressure wound therapy (NPWT) involves a portable device that removes wound fluids, stimulates the formation of granulation tissue, reduces bacteria growth, and helps draw wound edges together though the use of controlled negative pressure.

Indications: Clean (less than 20% necrotic/slough) chronic wounds, dehisced wounds, ulcers, surgical wounds, burns.

Advantages: Increases blood perfusion and nutrients to the wound tissue

Disadvantages: Pain, high cost, having to remember to turn the machine on, dressing seal leaks, application knowledge curve

Note: Inspect the machine daily, making sure that it is plugged in, settings are correct, and suction is working.

- A negative-pressure machine should not be off for more than 2 hours during a 24-hour period.

Treatment Protocol

- Gather supplies, premedicate the patient for pain and position the patient, remove the dressing, and cleanse the wound.
- Check orders; assess, measure, and take a photo of the wound. Reminder to date, sign, and place all documentation in the patient's chart.

Continued

Exhibit 12.4   *Continued*

- Apply a protective barrier and transparent drape to the periwound.
- Cut to size and apply the appropriate sponge to the wound bed (and tunneling/undermining).
- Apply a transparent dressing over the sponge to form an airtight seal.
- Attach a track pad to the transparent film dressing after cutting a hole in the film.
- Attach tubing to canister tubing, open clamps, and turn on the machine. Check settings.
- *Note:* Not all devices are the same. Compare facility guidelines with device instructions.

Side Effects: Bleeding

Contraindications: Wound with osteomyelitis, wound with malignant cells, necrotic tissue, the patient is on anticoagulants

Product Names: VAC™ by KCI, V.A.C. Via™

Exhibit 12.5   Pulsatile Lavage With Suction

Pulsatile Lavage With Suction

Definition: Pulsatile lavage with suction (PLWS) involves a pulsed irrigation device combined with suction that debrides, cleans, and irrigates a wound.

Indications: Wounds, burns needing debridement

Advantages: Can be used on infected wounds and wounds with necrotic tissue, promotes granulation	*Disadvantages:* Procedure learning curve, requires training, high cost

Continued

Exhibit 12.5 *Continued*

Note: Use protective apparel and clean the procedure area after treatment.

Treatment Protocol

- Only trained medical professionals should use this procedure.
- Check operating pressure and test it before starting the procedure.
- Use room-temperature normal saline.
- Premedicate the patient for pain.
- Treatments range from twice a day to 2 or 3 times a week.
- Follow guidelines per device instructions.

Side Effects: Bleeding, possible damage to other tissues, possible dissemination of bacteria

Contraindications: Patients on anticoagulants, patients who have neuropathy

Product Names: Pulsavac® by Zimmer, Simpulse® by VariCare

13

Caring for Ostomies and Fistulas

INTRODUCTION

Even dedicated, experienced, and specialized nurses in the field of ostomy management find the artificial openings and abnormal passageways of ostomies and fistulas overwhelming at times. Caring for ostomies and fistulas is a multifaceted, complex process. Every ostomy and fistula is as unique as the patient of whom it is a part. For the dedicated wound care nurse who seeks to expand his or her realm of expertise, it takes willingness and time to develop an expert knowledge base for the care of ostomies and fistulas. This chapter provides information about ostomies and fistulas that will encourage growth and enhance the knowledge of the dedicated wound care nurse.

In this chapter, you will learn:

1. The different etiologies of ostomies and fistulas, and some common complications.
2. The classification of ostomies and fistulas by location and complexity.
3. The types of products that are used in the care of ostomies and fistulas and how to use them, nutritional management, and methods of odor control.

177

OSTOMIES

An ostomy is an opening in the abdomen created by a surgical procedure for the elimination of body wastes. The incision is made through the abdominal wall. The end of the bowel is pulled through the opening and is then called a stoma. Stomas are not painful. Where the opening is made and how much of the intestines or bladder is removed dictate the kind of ostomy preformed. Don't be afraid of them.

There are three major kinds:

1. *Colostomy:* It may be temporary or permanent. It involves an opening in the large intestine (colon) for the elimination of stools. Loss of the rectum usually involves a permanent colostomy. After healing, stools are semi-formed to formed and brown in color.
2. *Ileostomy:* It may be temporary or permanent. It involves an opening in the small intestines to bypass the colon for the elimination of stools. The temporary alternative method is removal of the colon and rectum, creating an internal pouch from the small intestines to hold stools, attaching the pouch to the anus; this is called an ileoanal reservoir. Stools are green liquid at first, and later they are semi-formed and brownish.
3. *Urostomy:* This is a permanent bladder replacement for holding urine. An ileal loop or colon conduit is performed, using the end section of the small intestine (ileum) or the beginning of the large intestine (cecum), to form a stoma for urine to pass through.

Stoma Assessment

Bright red stomas indicate good circulation. New stomas are swollen and will shrink with time. A pink stoma may indicate that the patient is anemic. Gray or black stomas indicate that the blood supply to the bowel is compromised, and the surgeon should be notified. Although the stoma itself is moist, the skin surrounding the stoma should be clean, dry, and intact.

Stoma Measurement

The stoma should be measured at each pouch change. A template may be made from the wafer backing and used to cut future pouches. The wafer should be no more than an 1/8 of an inch larger than the stoma. Good hygiene and skin care are essential.

Common Stoma Complications

Ideally, stomas are marked by a wound, ostomy, and continence nurse (WOCN) or by the surgeon before surgery. Some common stoma complications post-surgery include:

- *Poor site:* When the stoma location has been surgically placed in the belt line, too close to a boney prominence or the umbilicus, or in skin creases, making management and pouching difficult.
- *Hernias:* Common with ostomies because the opening is made through the muscle to bring the stoma to the skin surface. Hernias also tend to recur.
- *Stoma necrosis:* Tissue death from poor circulation and lack of blood flow. The stoma may start to appear dark-red or purplish and then become black.
- *Retraction:* When the stoma withdraws back below the skin level.
- *Prolapse:* When the bowel expands through the stoma.

═══════════════════════*FAST FACTS in a NUTSHELL*

Colostomy Classification and Stoma Sites

- *Ascending colostomy*: The stoma is usually on the right side, and drainage is liquid or pasty.
- *Transverse colostomy*: The stoma is usually in the middle, and drainage is usually semi-solid with odor.

Continued

Continued

- *Descending colostomy*: The stoma is usually on the left side, and there are usually normal stools with odor.
- *Sigmoid colostomy*: The stoma is usually on the left side, and there are usually normal stools with odor.

Ileostomy Stoma Site

Ileostomy: The stoma site is usually on the lower right side, and drainage is liquid or paste-like.

The Pouching System

This is called an ostomy pouch and may be a one- or two-piece system. The two-piece system consists of a pouch to collect waste and a wafer to hold the pouch in place. The wafer should be cut to fit the stoma. The one-piece system has a wafer connected to the pouch. There are many varieties of pouches and wafers, so be realistic and keep it simple. The fewer products that the patient has to use, the better. If there is a problem with the pouch, this does not' necessarily mean that you need more products. Figure out what the problem is and fix it.

- Did you apply warmth and pressure to the wafer? It takes warmth and gentle pressure to seal the wafer to the skin.
- Have you observed the patient's abdomen as he or she moves from a lying to sitting position? The patient may need a more flexible pouch, such as a one-piece system or a pouch with convexity.
- Is the stoma flush or contracted? Do you need a pouch with more convexity?
- Does the patient have deep skin folds? Do these folds need to be filled with a paste or paste strip for a more secure seal?

- Can the patient see where the pouch is? Does the patient need to use a mirror?
- Is the pouch being emptied regularly? The seal will break if it is not emptied regularly or too much gas is present. Would a gas filter help?

Last but not least, the best advice that I ever received from a bona fide ostomy nurse was, "Don't be afraid to think." Passing that nugget of wisdom to you, I will add this: "Think outside the stoma."

Ostomy and Fistula Products, Actions, and Indications

All ostomies require that the patient wear an ostomy pouch for elimination of waste. This is related to the surgery bypassing the sphincter muscle, causing involuntary control of elimination.

Fistulas may be difficult to dress or pouch; however, protecting the skin is crucial. The specialty products shown in Table 13.1 aid in choosing and achieving an effective skin-management plan.

TABLE 13.1 Ostomy and Fistula Products	
Product	**Actions and Possible Problems to Watch for**
Barrier creams	Protect the skin and repel moisture. If they are oily, they will interfere with the pouch seal.
Paste (tube or strip form)	Makes the skin surface level. It acts as caulking for protection but will "melt out" with urine.

Continued

Product	Actions and Possible Problems to Watch for
Powder (ostomy)	Absorbs moisture from denuded skin and creates a scab layer. This is not an antifungal powder.
Pouches	The containers for effluent, stools, and odor.
Skin barrier sealants and wipes	Provide a smooth layer to allow the pouch to stick over powder; are helpful with iliostomies. Make sure the patient does not have allergies to these.
Skin barrier rings	Used as a level on concave skin surfaces; can be used in place of paste or to add convexity.
Solid wafers	Used to level the skin surface and to protect skin from effluent.

TABLE 13.1   Ostomy and Fistula Products *Continued*

==========*FAST FACTS in a NUTSHELL*

Basic Ostomy Pouch Guidelines

- *Supplies*: Water, nonsterile gauze, scissors, pouch with wafer, pattern, paste (if needed), and closure clip.
- Prepare the patient (position, remove pouch, clean the stoma and surrounding skin, measure the stoma and photograph if applicable). Fill in uneven areas, using strips or paste.
- Prepare the wafer by tracing the pattern on paper backing and cutting to fit, and then remove the paper backing. Snap the pouch on the ring if a two-piece

Continued

Continued

system is used. Apply a ring of paste around the stoma opening on the wafer of the pouch (like a ring of caulk). Do not spread the paste. Then apply the wafer.

- Control stoma drainage with gauze.
- Gently hold the pouch in place, giving it time to conform and seal.
- Close the bottom edge of the drainable pouch with a clamp or clampless closure. You may picture-frame the edges of the wafer with paper tape or waterproof tape.
- Document the procedure, color of stoma, condition of the skin, what is being eliminated (stool, gas, liquid), the patient's response, and education of patient/family.
- *Note:* For a new ostomy patient, have him or her assist with pouch changes as much as able or willing. For an established ostomy patient, let him or her tell you how he or she puts on the pouch. Patients are happy if you do it their way.

Ostomy Supplies and Medicare Limits

Reimbursement and coverage (such as Medicare) for ostomy supplies may vary. Take into consideration different insurers and different regional reimbursement policies. The information provided in Table 13.2 is not all inclusive.

FISTULAS

A fistula is an abnormal passageway that erupts through the surface of the skin, from an organ in the body, or from an abnormal communication from one hollow organ to another. An external fistula is named according to the

TABLE 13.2   Ostomy Supplies and Medicare Limits

Accessory Items	30 to 90 Day Supply	Product Suppliers	HCPCS Code
Adhesive liquid	4–12 oz	Hollister	A4364, A5120
Adhesive remover		Smith & Nephew	A4365, A4455
Pouch cleaner	1–3 bottles	Hollister	A5131
Belt	1–3 each	Coloplast/ ConvaTec/ Hollister/ NuHope	A4367
Catheter for continent stoma	1–3 each		
Convex Inserts	10–30 each	ConvaTec	A5093
Drain bag for urostomy	2–6 each	Bard	
Deodorizers		Anacapa/ Coloplast/ Hollister	A4394
Irrigation sleeve	4–2 each	Coloplast/ Hollister/ ConvaTec	A4397
Lubricant	4–12 oz	Coloplast/ ConvaTec/ Hollister	A4402

Continued

TABLE 13.2   Ostomy Supplies and Medicare Limits *Continued*

Accessory Items	30 to 90 Day Supply	Product Suppliers	HCPCS Code
Paste	4–12 oz	Coloplast/ ConvaTec/ Hollister	A4406, A4405
Pouch clamps		Coloplast/ ConvaTec/ Hollister	A4363
Powder (ostomy)	10–30 oz	Coloplast/ ConvaTec/ Hollister	A4371, A4371
Skin barrier	20–60 each	Coloplast/ ConvaTec/ Hollister	A5119, A4369
Skin barrier spray	2–6 oz	3M	A4369, A5120
Stoma cap	31–93 each	Austin/ Coloplast/ ConvaTec/ Hollister	A5055, A5083
Stoma plug for continent stoma	31–93 each	Hollister	A4368
Tape, nonwaterproof	40–120 units		
Tape, waterproof	40–120 units	Nu-Hope/ HyTape	A4452

Continued

TABLE 13.2   Ostomy Supplies and Medicare Limits *Continued*

Ostomy Pouches	30 to 90 Day Supply	Product Suppliers	HCPCS Code
Closed pouches • 1-Piece • 2-Piece • Preemie to pediatric	60–180 each	Coloplast/ Hollister/ Marlen/ ConvaTec	A4414, A4416 A5051, A4419 Babies: A4425, A5061, A5071, A5054
Drainable pouches • 1-Piece • 2-Piece	20–60 each	Coloplast/ ConvaTec/ Hollister	A4388, A4389, A5061, A4424, A4425, A5063, A4413
Urostomy pouches • 1-Piece • 2-Piece	20–60 each	Coloplast/ ConvaTec/ Hollister	A5073, A4432, A4421, A4428, A4393

Ostomy Wafers	30 to 90 Day Supply	Product Suppliers	HCPCS Code
Wafers Regular wear Extended wear	20–60 each	Coloplast/ ConvaTec/ Hollister	A4407, A4373, A4385, A4414, A4409

Note: These factors should influence your pouch selection: stoma size, shape, and location; the type, volume, and odor of drainage; skin integrity; patient ability and visual acuity; need for access; pouch wear time; and cost.

organ from which the drainage originates, such as a small bowel fistula or a pancreatic fistula. One of the most common ways to classify fistulas is as being either simple or complex:

- *Simple:* Short, direct, with no associated abscess or other organ involvement.
- *Complex:*
  - Type 1: Associated with abscess or multiple organs.
  - Type 2: On the surface; drains through the base of an open wound.

A fistula may also be classified as purposeful if it is created for a specific reason, or as inadvertent if it is a complication from disease, trauma, surgery, inflammation, or a congenital defect. One of the most common sites of origin for a fistula is a suture line, and the wound care nurse is often the first to recognize it through observations of changes in drainage (type, color, etc.).

═══════════════════════════*FAST FACTS in a NUTSHELL*

Anatomically Based Classification of Fistulas

- *Colocutaneous*: A passage between the colon and the skin.
- *Colovesical*: A fistula between the colon and the bladder.
- *Enterocutaneous*: A cutaneous fistula connecting the intestines and the skin.
- *Rectovaginal*: A fistula connecting the rectum and the vagina.
- *Vesicovaginal*: An abnormal connection between the bladder and the vagina.

Assessing Fistulas

Take your time in assessing fistulas. Thorough assessment and documentation will facilitate the best collaborative intervention choices for the patient from a multidisciplinary approach.

Location

Where is the fistula? Is it internal or external, close to an ostomy site, another opening, a wound, a surgical incision, a bony prominence, or is it in a concave area? Is there more than one?

Drainage (Figure 13.1)

Low volume is considered less than 200 mL/24 hr. High volume is considered over 200 mL/24 hr. The drainage from the stoma is called effluent. Note the consistency, color (gold, green, brown), and volume. The amount of drainage that is diverted from the fistula establishes whether it is a partial or complete fistula. Even a patient who takes nothing by mouth and has a nasogastric tube connected to suction may have an output of 2 to 3 liters of drainage per day.

Goal for a Plan of Management

1. Determine the amount of drainage.
2. Stabilize and maintain a positive nitrogen balance.
3. Stabilize and maintain fluid and electrolyte balance.
4. Give psychological support.

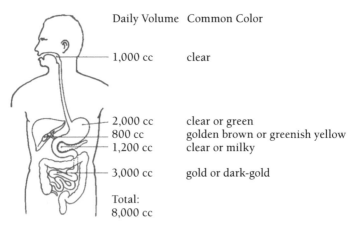

	Daily Volume	Common Color
	1,000 cc	clear
	2,000 cc	clear or green
	800 cc	golden brown or greenish yellow
	1,200 cc	clear or milky
	3,000 cc	gold or dark-gold
	Total: 8,000 cc	

FIGURE 13.1   Expected Drainage

Investigate the Cause

A computed tomography (CT) scan may be ordered to establish the origin of the fistula and condition of the adjacent bowel. The CT scan will also rule out possible obstruction and/or abscesses. These are factors that may lead to the development of a fistula (or delay of closure). Other factors may be Crohn's disease, previous radiation therapy, an inadequate blood supply, the presence of a tumor, the presence of a foreign body, abdominal trauma, or improper suturing. Take time to review the patient's history. Fistulas require frequent re-assessment and aggressive care. Can it be pouched? Choosing a pouch instead of a dressing allows more accurate measurement of drainage, protects the skin, is more comfortable for the patient, and is cost- effective because there is no continual changing of dressings, clothes, and linens. If pouching is not suitable, suction systems or V.A.C.™ therapy may be an appropriate option. Suction systems contain the effluent in combination with the dressing with low, intermittent suction. Consider V.A.C.™ therapy for the application of direct pressure closure.

Perifistular Skin

Assess the tissue surrounding the fistula. The secretions may be enzymatic and corrosive. Document the integrity of the tissue: Is it intact, denuded, and/or macerated, and are there signs of infection? Also assess the patient's pain.

Mortality Rates

Surgical complications remain the leading cause of fistula-related deaths. Infections, malnutrition, and fluid and electrolyte imbalances are fistula complications that can lead to death. Mortality rates vary between 5% and 20%. However, they are significantly lower with aggressive nutritional support.

Nutritional Management and Support

Nutritional therapy options may include:

- Electrolyte replacement, vitamin replacement, and rehydration (IV fluids).
- Nutritional support (total parenteral nutrition [TPN], fat emulsions, and enteral nutrition).
- Correcting anemia (blood replacement).
- Understanding what affects the consistency and amount of output.
- Eliminating foods that make the patient uncomfortable or make patient unable to take food by mouth (NPO) (Table 13.3).

Odor Assessment

Modern pouches are usually odor resistant. Good hygiene and cleaning equipment is essential for controlling odors (Table 13.4). Many products are available for additional odor control. Products are subject to personal preference, some working well for some patients with ostomies but not for others. For more information, contact a wound, ostomy, and continence nurse (WOCN). For information on where to locate a WOCN in your area, go to: http://www.wocn.org

Nursing and Patient Support

Nurse to Patient

The wound care nurse can and should offer support to patients. Patients are weak, tired, and fearful when it comes to coping with the physical strains of ostomies and fistulas. The wound care nurse can calm the patient by communicating about his or her status and treatment plans. Besides the ostomy, a patient's life may be complicated by pain, anxiety, poor body image, and the expenses of treatment.

TABLE 13.3 Foods That May Cause Gas, Odor, or Stool Thickening

Gas-Forming Foods	Odor-Producing Foods	Stool-Thickening Foods
asparagus, beer, broccoli, brussels sprouts, cabbage, carbonated drinks, corn, cucumbers, dairy products, dried beans, eggs, fish, garlic, melons, onions, radishes, spinach, sugars, sweet potatoes, sweets	asparagus, broccoli, brussels sprouts, cabbage, cauliflower, chicken, coffee, eggs, fish, garlic, onion, seafood	applesauce, bananas, boiled milk, bread, butter, cheese, creamy peanut butter, marshmallows, pasta, potatoes, pretzels, tapioca, tea, white bread, white rice

High-Fiber Foods	Odor-Reducing Foods	Foods That Control Mild Constipation
popcorn, nuts, coconuts, tomatoes, mushrooms, raw apples, strawberries, grapes, pineapple, raw coleslaw, salad greens, celery, cooked spinach, green beans, and corn	buttermilk, cranberry juice, parsley, yogurt	cooked fruits and vegetables, fruit juices, fluids

Note: Certain foods such as beets, red gelatin desserts, and red velvet cake will color stools.

TABLE 13.4   Odor Control Options

Colostomies and Ileostomies	Urinary Diversions
External-Use Products	**External-Use Products**
Disinfectant Room Sprays: Spraying the room with disinfectant when changing a pouch is helpful. (Examples: Lysol, Medi-Aire Air Freshener, Odor Eliminator) *Deodorants:* Deodorants come in the form of liquids or tablets that can be added to the pouch; these may be the most expensive option but are the most effective. (Examples: Banish, M-9 Drop Deodorizer) *Mild Soaps:* Using several squirts of a mild soap with or without mouthwash when the pouch is first applied and each time it is emptied and rinsed reduces odor. (Examples: Remedy, Aloe Vesta, Uniwash) *Mouthwash:* A small amount of any preferred mouthwash in the pouch is a simple and inexpensive method of odor control.	*Pouch Cleaners:* These may facilitate the elimination of urine odor in two-piece pouches that are reused. Remember to use cool water when cleaning pouches and using these products. (Examples: Urolux, Urikleen, or any perineal soaps)
Oral Medications	**Oral Medications**

Note: All oral medications should be discussed with the physician, even when they are available without a prescription.

Bismuth Subgallate: Devrom chewable tablets taken at meals and bedtime starts odor control before it reaches the pouch. *Chlorophyllin Copper Complex:* One or two Nullo tablets taken three times a day before meals helps with odor control.	*Vitamin C 500 mg:* Tablets taken 3 to 4 times a day will help control odors and also may help control urinary tract infections.

Nurse to Nurse

Get to know your local WOCNs and certified wound specialists (CWSs). Most of them are more than willing to offer support, feedback, and encouragement when it comes to their expertise in wounds and ostomies. They can make a significant difference in your patients' outcomes.

FAST FACTS in a NUTSHELL

Helpful Ostomy Organizations

- Crohn's and Colitis Foundation of America, Inc.: 800-932-2423
- Evansville Ostomy News Hints and Tips: http://www.ostomy.evansville.net/hints.htm
- International Foundation for Functional Gastrointestinal Disorders: 414-964-1799, http://www.iffgd.org
- The National Digestive Diseases Clearinghouse: 800-891-5389, http://digestive.niddk.nih.gov
- The Wound, Ostomy, and Continence Nurse Society (WOCNS): 888-224-9626, http://www.wocn.org
- The United Ostomy Association of America (UOAA): 800-826-0826, http://www.ostomy.org
- The Young Ostomate and Diversion Alliance of America (YODAA): www.yodaa.org

Note: I would like to express my deep thanks to Camille Spess, WOCN, MS, RN, ET Nurse, whose profound influence has contributed significantly to this chapter.

14

The Promotion of Skin Care Integrity

INTRODUCTION

Why is skin care so important? The skin is the largest organ of the body and performs major functions, such as absorption from respiration, control of evaporation, heat regulation, protection from pathogens, sensation communication, water resistance, and metabolism. By performing these functions, the skin protects the bones, internal organs, ligaments, and muscles.

However, the skin's characteristics are constantly changing in response to environmental, chemical, and physical factors, such as the sun, age, hydration, nutrition, medications, and skin care products. If the skin's integrity is jeopardized, a person's skin function may be at risk. Practical assessment, appropriate care, and perceptive prevention are the keys to promoting optimum skin care integrity.

In this chapter, you will learn:

1. Factors that affect skin integrity.
2. How to perform a skin assessment.
3. About FDA approval, categories, and manufacturers of skin care products.
4. Why incontinence maintenance is the foundation of a successful skin and wound care program.

195

FACTORS THAT AFFECT SKIN INTEGRITY

- *Aging:* The aging process can decrease all the normal functions of the skin over time.
- *Allergies:* Allergies are caused by irritants that can lead to itching, skin rashes, pain, and sores.
- *Circulation:* Poor circulation can lead to ulceration. For the skin to receive good blood flow, sufficient blood volume must flow through unclogged arteries and veins, via an adequately regulated heart, providing sufficient capillary refill. Review patients' history for previous ulcers.
- *Hydration:* Poor hydration can cause dry, cracked, scaly skin. Besides a lack of fluids, humidity, age, and lost sebum contribute to poor hydration. Moisturizers are advantageous.
- *Lifestyle Habits:* Poor hygiene can lead to skin infections, and smoking affects circulation.
- *Medications:* Medications such as corticosteroids can cause thinning of skin related to interference with collagen synthesis and epidermal regeneration. Anticoagulants may cause bruising. Some medications may even cause the skin to slough.
- *Nutrition:* Poor nutrition can lead to skin breakdown. A well-balanced diet of proteins, carbohydrates, fats, vitamins, and minerals is essential for healthy skin. Patients who are experiencing complex skin breakdown, such as a burn, require increased dietary intake.
- *Soaps:* Normal bathing restores skin pH. However, harsh chemicals in some soaps used over a long period of time can impair the skin's resistance to bacteria and its water-holding capacity.
- *Sun Exposure:* Excessive sun exposure decreases skin elasticity, causes wrinkling, and can lead to cancer related to ultraviolet radiation (UVR) damage.

SKIN ASSESSMENT

A head-to-toe skin assessment should be performed on every patient upon admission. Commonly missed areas are behind the ears, between the toes, the heels, the back of the head, and under skin folds. A practical skin assessment can give the nurse realistic indicators of the patient's condition, circulation status, and healing ability. Skin integrity may be difficult and challenging with sick, compromised patients. Performing a basic skin car assessment is crucial to implementing appropriate care.

Skin Assessment Indicators

- *Capillary Refill:* An indicator of blood perfusion at the capillary level.
- *Color:* White, pale, ashy, waxy skin may be an indicator of poor peripheral circulation, a deep burn, or frostbite. Blue or gray skin is an indicator of cyanosis. Red skin may be an indicator of fever, mild burns, or carbon-monoxide poisoning. Yellow skin may be an indicator of liver disease. Also check the nail beds, mucous membranes, and whites of the eyes.
- *Integrity:* Check the overall health of the skin, observing any fragility, bruising, skin tears, excoriation, denuded skin, decreased sensation, edema, wounds, old scars, and healed ulcer sites.
- *Moisture:* Excessively dry or clammy and sticky skin may be an indicator of underlying disease processes.
- *Poor Hygiene:* A strong odor may be an indicator of infection.
- *Temperature:* Normal skin is warm to the touch. Skin that is hot to the touch may be an indicator of fever, hyperthermia, inflammation, or a mild burn. Skin that is cold to the touch may be an indicator of poor circulation, early shock, hypothermia, or frostbite.
- *Turgor:* Skin with normal turgor springs back to a normal position after it has been pinched. Decreased turgor may be an indicator of dehydration.

================*FAST FACTS in a NUTSHELL*

Skin Care Products

Are your skin care products approved by the U.S. FDA? As a patient advocate, it is important for you to understand that under federal law, the products that you apply to your patients may be FDA approved as a cosmetic, drug, soap, or a combination of these, or it may not be FDA approved at all. FDA approval plays an important role in assuring the nurse that a product has not been adulterated or misbranded. The FDA categorizes drugs, soaps, and cosmetics by their intended use. There are multiple ways in which the FDA establishes the intended use of a product based on its ingredients, such as regulating claims on product labels, in advertising, and on the Internet. For more information on the FDA's skin care product approval criteria, go to: http://www.fda.gov.

Common Skin Care Formulary Options

Cleansers

Cleansers are used for bathing and for removing surface dirt, impurities, perspiration, and excessive oils. Bathing with advanced cleansers also help rehydrate and nourish skin.

Topical Antifungals

Antifungal medication in powder or cream form is used to treat skin infections, usually caused by trichophyton, epidermophyton, or microsporum.

Moisturizers

Moisturizers come in different formulations. Understanding the differences among lotions, creams, and ointments is

TABLE 14.1   Skin Care Product Options (Not All Inclusive)

Skin and Incontinence Cleansers

Bottled Bathing Products	Disposable Bathing Products	Incontinence Cleaners
Remedy 4-in-1 by Medline	ReadyBath by Medline	Elta® by Swiss-American
Secura ™ by Smith & Nephew	Aloe Vesta® by ConvaTec	Aloe Vesta® Foam by ConvaTec
Elta® by Swiss-American	Attends Washcloths® by 3M	Restore® by Hollister
ApriVera® by Derma Sciences	Baza Cleanse & Protect by Coloplast	Bedside-Care® by Coloplast
Gentle Rain® by Coloplast	Comfort Bath® by Sage	Aloe Vesta® by ConvaTec
Septi-Soft® by ConvaTec		Soothe & Cool® by Medline
Cavilon™ Skin Cleanser by 3M		Secura™ by Smith & Nephew

Topical Antifungals

Creams	Ointments	Powders
Remedy by Medline	Aloe Vesta® by ConvaTec	Remedy by Medline
Micro-Guard® by Coloplast	DermaFungal by DermaRite	MITRAZOL® by Healthpoint
Baza® by Coloplast	Critic-Aid® by Coloplast	Micro-Guard® by Coloplast

Continued

TABLE 14.1   Skin Care Product Options (Not All Inclusive) *Continued*

Topical Antifungals

Creams	Ointments	Powders
INZO™ by Medline	Aloe Vesta® by ConvaTec	
	Elta® Trivase by Swiss-American	

Moisturizers

Creams	Ointments	Zinc-Oxide Barriers
Sensi-Care® Cream by ConvaTec	Aloe Vesta® by ConvaTec	Sensi-Care® by ConvaTec
Uni-Derm® by Smith & Nephew	Secura™ by Smith & Nephew	Secura™ by Smith & Nephew
Cavilon™ Emollient by 3M	Restore® Ointment by Hollister	Bacitracin Zinc by Dynarex
Eucerin® Cream by Beiersdorf	Calmoseptine® by Calmoseptine	
Hydrocortisone Cream by Dynarex	Aquaphor® Ointment by Beiersdorf	
	Baza® by Coloplast	

important when choosing the most appropriate product for a particular need.

- *Lotions:* Good for normal to mildly dry skin. Lotions are made with oils, usually mixed in a low-viscosity water base that is easily absorbed into the skin.
- *Creams:* Good for moderately to very dry skin and also to help prevent skin cracking or tears. Creams are emulsified oils, usually mixed in a high-viscosity water base.
- *Ointment:* Good for moisture protection and also to help remove thick, dead skin on the heels and feet. Ointments are very viscous, semisolid preparations and usually have an occlusive oil base. Ointments are good emollients for active ingredients in topicals.
- *Zinc-Oxide Barrier:* Good as a moisture barrier for excoriated skin resulting from feces or urine, and/or other skin irritations. Zinc-oxide powder is added to an assortment of cream bases. Zinc oxide provides a moisture barrier over painful, raw skin.

Choose skin care products carefully. Skin care integrity is the foundation of a successful wound and skin care program.

FECAL AND BLADDER INCONTINENCE

According to the National Association for Continence (NAFC), 13 million Americans are incontinent, and 85% of these are women. These data, combined with the fact that moisture is one of the predisposing factors in pressure ulcer development, make a good skin care program high on the health care priority list. Incontinence may be caused by many factors, including stress, surgery, decreased sensation, severe diarrhea, or chronic laxative abuse.

==*FAST FACTS in a NUTSHELL*

Types of Incontinence

- *Anatomic Incontinence*: Leakage caused by an anatomic or neurologic abnormality, such as a fistula.
- *Bed Wetting*: Considered normal in children until the age of 5.
- *Fecal Incontinence*: A loss of normal control of the bowel.
- *Functional Incontinence*: Most common in the elderly because of an inability to control the bladder related to time and limitations in moving, thinking, and/or communicating. It may be caused by disease processes (e.g., Parkinson's or Alzheimer's disease).
- *Mixed Incontinence*: The experiencing by a person (usually a woman) of more than one type of incontinence.
- *Overflow Incontinence*: Urination triggered by a bladder that does not' completely empty. A constantly full bladder may lead to weak muscles, causing dribbling.
- *Stress Incontinence*: An involuntary leak related to coughing, laughing, sneezing, or pressure-related activities.
- *Temporary Incontinence*: Temporary leakage may be a side effect of various medical conditions, such as severe constipation, an infection, or medications.
- *Urge Incontinence*: May be known as reflex, spastic, or overactive bladder and is caused by a sudden, uncontrollable urge to urinate. This may happen while a person is sleeping or hears a trigger such as running water.

FACILITY NAME and LOGO
Policy/Procedure Manual

Policy/Procedure

Number:
Page:
Prepared by:
Date:

Scope: Nursing Personnel

Subject: Skin-Care Guidelines: Cleanse, Moisturize, and Protect

Purpose: To decrease discrepancies and to promote appropriate and efficient care

Policy: Intervention to prevent breakdown, and promote and restore healthy skin

Procedure: Techniques, instructions, and steps

1. Inspect the skin daily, noting any changes, such as reddened areas, deep tissue injury, bruises, blisters, skin tears, and/or wounds.
2. Gather supplies for bathing using a minimum of 8 to 9 washcloths. Each cloth will be used for a different area of the body, reducing cross-contamination (one each for the face and neck, the chest, each arm/axilla, each leg, the perineum, the back, and the buttocks). Towels, pH-balanced soap, moisturizer, clean clothing, and linens are also needed.
3. Start from the top, placing a warmed shampoo cap on the patient.
4. Proceed downward, undressing the top half of body, washing, patting dry, applying deodorant and moisturizer, and redressing the patient. Cover the top half of the body with clean linens.
5. Proceed downward, undressing the lower half of body, washing, patting dry, moisturizing (applying a protectant or barrier, if appropriate), and redressing the patient. Pull clean linens down over the lower part of the body.
6. Massage the patient's scalp with the shampoo cap still in place. Remove the cap, rinse the hair, and gently dry it. Comb the hair. Perform oral care.

FIGURE 14.1   Bathing Guidelines

Continued

Continued

7. Reposition the patient according to the turn clock position. Protect bony prominences. Position the heels off the bed, using pillows for support.
8. Document the procedure, patient tolerance, and the turn clock position.

| | Effective Date: | Approved by: |
| Supersedes Policy Dated: | Prepared by: | Approved by: |

FIGURE 14.1   Bathing Guidelines

Types of Incontinence Products

There are numerous products to assist with incontinence, giving people various options related to their lifestyles and better quality of life. Such products include but are not limited to breathable under pads, protective underwear, belted undergarments, liners, pads, and disposable briefs. In the intensive care setting, fecal management systems may be used, such as the Zassi™ Bowel Management System or the ConvaTec Flexi-Seal® System. The use of these systems requires in-service education and an understanding of indication warnings for patient selection.

However, a bath—a nurse's labor of caring—may be the most meaningful option. Bathing not only cleanses the body, but it also reduces body odor, provides exercise, stimulates circulation, and even improves self-image. It may seem old fashioned in the high-tech world we live in, but evidence-based practice still considers bathing the best means for skin healing. Figure 14.1 shows a policy/procedure template for bathing guidelines.

FAST FACTS in a NUTSHELL

Prevention Awareness Tips for Optimal Skin Care

- Use lots of pillows as a cost-efficient way to support the patient's position and separate bony prominences.
- Educate the patient and family about prevention awareness.
- Enforce a 2-hour (or less) turn schedule.
- Float the patient's heels off the bed using pillows to support the calves and knees.
- Keep the head of the bed at 30-degree angle° (or less) if appropriate.
- Keep the patient clean and dry (change linens and gown as needed).
- Moisturize the patient's skin often to strengthen and protect it.
- Prevent sheering on the patient's toes by untucking the covers over the feet and making a tent, using a foot cradle.
- Protect the patient's limbs from bed rails by covering the rails with padding (e.g., towels taped on the rails).
- Remind a sitting patient to shift positions every 15 minutes.
- Use appropriate draw sheet, trapeze, and bariatric devices when turning the patient.

Skin Care Education for Patients and Family Members

Supply the patient with any necessary or helpful phone numbers and emphasize to him or her the importance of skin care. Instruct the patient to do the following:

- Don't be afraid to seek help, ask questions, or explain your needs and wants.

- Keep yourself and your environment clean and dry. Involve family members and caregivers if necessary.
- Eat a well-balanced diet. Healing requires good nutrition.
- Exercise or increase your activity level to promote good circulation.
- Check your skin daily. Notify your physician of any of the following: signs of infection, new wounds, skin condition changes (customize this information for each individual patient).

15

Selecting Optimal Support Surfaces and Equipment for Patient Positioning

INTRODUCTION

In the past, bed frames were strung with ropes. Today, a patient bed is a specialized device known as a support surface, with pressure redistribution being the ultimate goal. Choosing a patient's support surface to prevent or care for pressure ulcers can be as critical as the diagnosis, and the support surface can be even more costly. In 2007, Medicare payments for support surfaces totaled $137 million, $118 million of which was for rentals. Those amounts represent only the claims that were paid. The amount of money spent on support surfaces is just as staggering today, and so is the complexity of support surfaces. They range from reactive supports to active supports, integrated bed systems, non-powered beds, powered beds, and overlays to simple standard mattresses. Although the support surface is only one part of a comprehensive treatment plan, it can be crucial to a patient's outcome.

In this chapter, you will learn:

1. NPUAP categories, mechanical characteristics, components, and physical concepts of support surfaces.
2. Factors that guide the selection of a support surface.
3. Advantages and disadvantages of support system surfaces.
4. About bariatric equipment.
5. Centers for Medicare and Medicaid Services (CMS) support surface guidelines and coding information.

SUPPORT SURFACES

The CMS and the National Pressure Ulcer Advisory Panel (NPUAP) address support surfaces. Qualifying support surface criteria is essential to choosing the most appropriate surface for the patient and to providing the greatest cost savings to the facility. The NPUAP provides the best-respected evidence-based nursing research available on support surfaces, and CMS guidelines are the most standardized for addressing coverage of support surfaces.

The CMS classifies support surfaces into three categories: pressure pads and mattress overlays, special rented mattresses placed over bed frames, and special bed systems. The NPUAP and CMS work together to develop consistent terminology so that standards are uniform.

═══════════════════════════*FAST FACTS in a NUTSHELL*

The National Pressure Ulcer Advisory Panel (NPUAP) defines a *support surface* as "a specialized device for pressure redistribution designed for management of tissue loads, micro-climate, and/or other therapeutic functions (i.e., any mattresses, integrated bed system, mattress replacement, overlay, or seat cushion, or seat cushion overlay."

TABLE 15.1   NPUAP Categories and Mechanical Characteristics of Support Surfaces

Support Surface	Definition
Reactive Support Surface	A powered or non-powered support surface with the capability to change its load distribution properties only in response to an applied load.
Active Support Surface	A powered support surface with the capability to change its load distribution properties with or without an applied load.
Integrated Bed System	A bed frame and support surface that are combined into a single unit whereby the surface is unable to function separately.
Non-powered Support Surface (historically called a static support surface)	Any support surface not requiring or using external sources of energy for operation. (Energy = D/C or A/C)
Powered Support Surface (historically called dynamic)	Any support surface requiring or using external sources of energy to operate. (Energy = D/C or A/C)
Overlay	An additional support surface designed to be placed directly on top of an existing surface.
Mattress	A support surface designed to be placed directly on the existing bed frame.

Functional features of a support surface may be used alone or in combination with others.

Table 15.2 NPUAP Features of Support Surfaces	
Features of Support Surface	Definition
Air Fluidizing	A feature of a support surface that provides pressure redistribution via a fluid-like medium created by forcing air through microsphere beads, as characterized by immersion and envelopment.
Alternating Pressure	A feature of a support surface that provides pressure redistribution via cyclic changes in loading and unloading, as characterized by frequency, duration, amplitude, and rate of change parameters.
Lateral Rotation	A feature of a support surface that provides rotation about a longitudinal axis, as characterized by degree of a patient's turn, duration, and frequency.
Low Air Loss	A feature of a support surface that provides a flow of air to assist in managing the heat and humidity (microclimate) of the skin.
Zone	A segment with a single pressure redistribution capability.
Multi-Zoned	A surface in which different segments can have different pressure redistribution capabilities.

Factors Guiding Selection of a Support Surface

- *The Patient:* No person is free from pressure because no person is weightless. Does the patient need more surface area, need the contact with the surface to be temporarily removed, or need contact shifted to other areas?
- *Weight and Height of the Patient:* Does the patient need a bariatric-sized bed?
- *Multiple Devices:* Is more than one device needed? For example, a morbidly obese patient needing a bariatric bed might also need a lift and bariatric bedside commode.
- *Tolerance:* Is the patient comfortable and pain free regarding the support surface?
- *Independent Functioning:* Some support surfaces interfere with the patient's ability to move off the bed. How high does the surface make the bed?
- *Compliance:* Most surfaces still require that patients be turned. Do the patient, staff, and family understand the importance of turning and repositioning?
- *Time:* Is the support surface needed for short-term or long-term (acute versus chronic) usage?
- *Feasibility:* Have the staff, family, and patient had proper in-service education about and are capable of performing equipment function?
- *Equipment Needs:* Is the room large enough for staff to work around the bed? Does it have working outlets, and are they placed in convenient locations for the bed?
- *Reimbursement:* Is the support surface financially feasible? Is there a contract already established with the facility?

========== *FAST FACTS in a NUTSHELL*

Indications for Various Support Surfaces

Existing Pressure Ulcer Patients: Is there a risk for development of additional pressure ulcers? Use a pressure-reducing surface if the patient remains at risk.

Non-powered (Static) Support Surface: Use if the patient can change positions without bearing weight on a pressure ulcer and without "bottoming out."

Powered (Dynamic) Support Surface: Use if the patient cannot change positions without bearing weight on a pressure ulcer, if the patient fully compresses the static support surface, or if the pressure ulcer does not show evidence of healing within 2 to 4 weeks.

Low-Air-Loss and Air-Fluidized Beds: Use if the patient had postoperative flap surgery, had large Stage III or IV pressure ulcers on multiple turning surfaces, bottoms out, or fails to heal on a powered overlay mattress.

Even using the guidelines above, how do you know which support surface to choose for your patient? The information in Figure 15.3 can help you with your selection. Components of a support surface may be used alone or in combination with others.

Bariatric Equipment Reality Check

Long gone are the days when draw sheets, gate belts, and even slide boards were sufficient tools for lifting, transferring, and repositioning patients. To be considered obese, a patient weighs at least 100 pounds more than his or her ideal body weight (IBW) or has a 40% higher body mass index (BMI). Obesity has continued to trend upward for the last 20 years. Patients weighing 300 pounds and more are not uncommon today. With 75% of Americans being overweight,

Table 15.3   NPUAP Components of Support Surfaces

Component	Definition
Air	A low-density fluid with minimal resistance to flow.
Cell/Bladder	A means of encapsulating a support medium.
Viscoelastic Foam (Memory Foam)	A type of porous polymer material that conforms in proportion to the applied weight. The air exists and enters the foam cells slowly, which allows the material to respond more slowly than standard elastic foam.
Elastic Foam (Non-memory Foam)	A type of porous polymer material that conforms in proportion to the applied weight. Air enters and exits the foam cells rapidly because of high density.
Closed Cell Foam	A non-permeable structure in which there is a barrier between cells, preventing gases or liquids from passing through the foam.
Open Cell Foam	A permeable structure in which there is no barrier between cells, and gases or liquids can pass through the foam.
Gel	A semisolid system consisting of a network of solid aggregates and colloidal dispersions or polymers, which may exhibit elastic properties. (Can range from a hard gel to a soft gel.)
Pad	A cushion-like mass of soft material used for comfort, protection or positioning.
Viscous Fluid	A fluid with a relatively high resistance to flow.
Elastomer	Any material that can be repeatedly stretched to at least twice its original length; upon release, the stretch will return to approximately its original length.
Solid	A substance that does not flow perceptibly under stress. Under ordinary conditions, it retains its size and shape.
Water	A moderate-density fluid with moderate resistance to flow.

Table 15.4   Advantages and Disadvantages of Support System Surfaces

Surface	Advantages	Disadvantages
Foam	Lightweight, one-time charge, resists puncture, many sizes, low maintenance	Retains heat, often thrown away when unprotected from drainage, retains moisture, limited life, fire hazard
Gel-Filled	Low maintenance, easy to clean, multiple-patient use, resists puncture	Heavy, expensive
Fluid-Filled	Easy to clean, baffle system available	Requires a heater, can leak, can be overfilled or underfilled, heavy, transfers are difficult
Air-Fluidized	Easy to clean, less patient turning is needed, multiple-patient use, low maintenance	Hot, heavy, expensive, noisy, requires regular monitoring for proper inflation, transfers are difficult
Low-Air-Loss	Requires less patient turning, easy to clean, maintains constant inflation, setup is provided by manufacturer	Requires power, restricts mobility, skilled setup required, noisy, expensive
Dynamic Overlays	Easy to clean, deflates for transfers, reusable pump, multiple-patient use	Assembly required, requires power
Mattress Replacements	Multiple-patient use, low maintenance, inexpensive options, reduces staff time	Requires power, initial expense is high, life of product may not be known, may not control moisture

Table 15.5 NPUAP Physical Concepts Related to Support Surfaces

Physical Concept	Definition
Friction (Frictional Force)	The resistance to motion in a parallel direction relative to the common boundary of two surfaces.
Coefficient of Friction	A measurement of the amount of friction existing between two surfaces.
Envelopment	The ability of a support surface to conform, so as to fit or mold around irregularities in the body.
Fatigue	The reduced capacity of a surface or its components to perform as specified. This change may be the result of intended or unintended use and/or prolonged exposure to chemical, thermal, or physical forces.
Force	A push–pull vector with magnitude (quantity) and direction (pressure, shear) that is capable of maintaining or altering the position of a body.
Immersion	The depth of penetration (sinking) into a support surface.
Life Expectancy	The defined period of time during which a product is able to effectively fulfill its designated purpose.
Mechanical Load	Force distribution acting on a surface.
Pressure	The force per unit area exerted perpendicular to the plane of interest.

Continued

Table 15.5 NPUAP Physical Concepts Related to Support Surfaces *Continued*

Physical Concept	Definition
Pressure Redistribution	The ability of a support surface to distribute a load over the contact areas of the human body. This term replaces prior terminology of *pressure reduction* and *pressure relief.*
Pressure Reduction	This term is no longer used to describe classes of support surfaces. The term used now is *pressure redistribution*; see above.
Pressure Relief	This term is no longer used to describe classes of support surfaces. The term used now is *pressure redistribution*; see above.
Shear (Shear Stress)	The force per unit area exerted parallel to the plane of interest.
Shear Strain	Distortion or deformation of tissue as a result of shear stress.

it should not be surprising that nurses have the highest injury claim rates of any occupation. More than one-third of nurses have back injuries related to manually lifting and transferring patients. Bariatric equipment may seem expensive initially, but is it in the long run? It is time to weigh the cost of nursing injuries (and shortages) versus the cost of bariatric equipment.

There are many bariatric options to choose from:

- *Ambulatory Assistance:* Canes, crutches, and walkers (KCI, Medline).
- *Assessment:* Scales (Medline).

- *Bathing:* Bath benches, shower benches, and shower chairs (KCI, Medline).
- *Beds:* There are a variety and ranges, such as cardio-chair position beds, overlay mattresses, and low-air-loss beds up to 54 inches wide that can bear 1,000 pounds of weight (Hill-Rom, KCI, Medline, Span-America Medical).

  Powered Beds: There are a variety and ranges, such as air-fluidized beds, low-air-loss beds, pulmonary beds, silver technology beds, beds with removable head and foot boards, turn-assist beds that can bear 700 pounds of weight and are 84 inches in length (Hill-Rom, KCI, Medline).

  Mattresses: Powered and non-powered mattresses and overlays (EHOB, Encompass Therapeutic Support Systems, KCI, Hill-Rom, Medline, Southwest, Talley Medical).

- *Furniture:* There are a variety and ranges, such as over-bed tables (Medline).
- *Incontinence:* There are a variety and ranges, such as briefs and bedside commodes (KCI, Medline).
- *Pressure Redistribution and Support:* There are a variety and ranges such as platforms, boots, elbow protectors, wedges, and rolls (Briggs, EHOB, DM Systems, Medline, Southwest, Talley).
- *Sitting:* There are a variety and ranges, such as chairs, cushions, recliners, and lifts (EHOB, Encompass Therapeutic Support Systems, Span-America Medical Systems, KCI, Medline, Talley).
- *Transporting:* Lifts, stretchers, transfer benches, and wheelchairs (Encompass Therapeutic Support Systems, Hill-Rom, KCI, Medline).

Taking into consideration bariatric equipment and understanding NPUAP support surface definitions will make it easier to choose a support surface using the CMS guidelines.

Exhibit 15.1   CMS Support Surface Guidelines

Group 1 Support Surfaces: These surfaces are designed to be placed on top of a standard hospital or home mattress. They include pressure pads and mattress (foam, air, water, or gel) overlays. They may be rented or purchased.

Patient Criteria for Group 1 Support Surfaces: The patient must meet one of the following criteria:
1. The patient is immobile (bedfast), unable to change positions, and requires assistance.
2. The patient is at risk of developing pressure ulcers related to limited mobility and has one of the following conditions:
   • Impaired nutritional status
   • Incontinence: fecal or urinary
   • Altered sensory perception
   • Compromised circulatory status
3. The patient has a staged pressure ulcer on the trunk or pelvis and one of the conditions listed above.

Note: For items 2 and 3, documentation must state the severity of the patient's condition that requires a support surface.

Coding Information
A4640: Replacement pad for use with medically necessary alternating pressure pad owned by the patient.
A9270: A non-covered item or service.
E0181: A powered, pressure-reducing mattress overlay/pad, alternating, with a pump, including those that are heavy duty. E0182: A pump for an alternating-pressure pad, for replacement only.
E0184: A dry pressure mattress.
E0185: A gel or gel-like pressure pad for a mattress, of standard mattress length and width.

Continued

Continued

E0186: An air-pressure mattress.

E0187: A water-pressure mattress.

E0188: A synthetic sheepskin pad.

E0189: A sheepskin pad, any size.

E0196: A gel-pressure mattress.

E0197: An air-pressure pad for a mattress of standard length and width.

E0198: A water-pressure pad for a mattress of standard length and width.

E0199: A dry-pressure pad for a mattress of standard length and width.

E1399: Durable medical equipment, miscellaneous.

The *Healthcare Common Procedure Coding System* (HCPCS) Modifiers: A support surface claim that does not meet the Coding Guideline requirements will be denied.

EY: There is no physician or other licensed health care provider order for the item.

GA: A waiver of liability statement is on file.

GZ: An item or service is expected to be denied as not reasonable and necessary.

KX: Requirements specified in the medical policy have been met.

═══════════════════════*FAST FACTS in a NUTSHELL*

Bottoming Out

Bottoming out is the finding that an outstretched hand, placed palm up between the undersurface of the mattress and the patient's bony prominence (coccyx or lateral trochanter), can readily palpate the bony prominence. Test and document with the patient in a supine position with the head flat, and again in a supine position with the head slightly elevated, and also in a side-lying position.

Continued

Group 2 Support Surfaces: These are special mattress overlays used alone or placed over a bed frame. They include air-flotation beds, powered pressure-reducing air mattresses, and non-powered advanced pressure-reducing mattresses. They are usually only rented and are more expensive than group 1 support surfaces.

Patient Criteria for Group 2 Support Surfaces: The patient must meet criteria 1, 2, and 3, or 4, or 5 and 6:
1. Multiple Stage II pressure ulcers are located on the trunk or pelvis (ICD-9 707.02–707.05)
2. The patient has been on a comprehensive ulcer treatment program for at least the past month, which has included the use of an appropriate Group 1 support surface.
3. The ulcers have worsened or remained the same over the past month.
4. Large or multiple Stage III or IV pressure ulcer(s) are located on the trunk or pelvis (ICD-9 707.02–707.05).
5. A recent mycutaneous flap or skin graft for a pressure ulcer is located on the trunk or pelvis (surgery within the past 60 days) (ICD-9 707.02–707.05).
6. The patient has been on a Group 2 or 3 support surface prior to discharge from a hospital or nursing facility (discharge within the past 30 days).

Coding Information
E0193: A powered pressure-reducing air mattress.
E0371: A non-powered advanced pressure-reducing overlay for a mattress of standard length and width.

Continued

Continued

E0372: A powered air overlay for a mattress of standard length and width.

E0373: A non-powered advanced pressure-reducing mattress.

E1399: Durable medical equipment, miscellaneous.

HCPCS Modifiers A support surface claim that does not meet the Coding Guideline requirements will be denied.

EY: There is no physician or other licensed health care provider order for the item.

GA: A waiver of liability statement is on file.

GZ: An item or service is expected to be denied as not reasonable and necessary.

KX: Requirements specified in the medical policy have been met.

Group 3 Support Surfaces: These are complete air-fluidized bed systems. They are usually only rented and more expensive than Group 2 support surfaces.

Patient Criteria for Group 3 Support Surfaces The patient must meet the following criteria:

1. The patient has a Stage III or IV pressure ulcer.
   - A Stage III or IV pressure ulcer of the foot does not require an air-fluidized bed because the foot can be elevated to relieve pressure.
   - If the patient is on an air-fluidized bed and an ulcer is less than 8 square centimeters and/or it is in an area other than the posterior trunk or pelvis, the attending physician must document why an alternative support surface would not be medically effective.
2. The patient is immobile or chair-bound as a result of severely limited mobility.

Continued

Continued

3. In the absence of an air-fluidized bed, the patient would require hospitalization or placement in a nursing home.
4. The air-fluidized bed is ordered in writing by the attending physician based upon a comprehensive assessment and evaluation of the patient after conservative treatment has been tried without success.
5. The evaluation generally must be performed within a week prior to initiation of therapy with the air-fluidized bed.
6. A trained adult caregiver is available to assist the patient with activities of daily living, fluid balance, dry skin care, repositioning, recognition and management of altered mental status, dietary needs, prescribed treatments, and management and support of the air-fluidized bed system and its problems, such as leakage.
7. A physician directs the home-treatment regimen and re-evaluates and re-certifies the need for the air-fluidized bed on a monthly basis.
8. All other alternative equipment has been considered and ruled out.

Coding Information
E0194: An air-fluidized bed.
HCPCS Modifiers: A support surface claim that does not meet the Coding Guideline requirements will be denied.
EY: There is no physician or other licensed health care provider order for the item.
GA: A waiver of liability statement is on file.
GZ: An item or service is expected to be denied as not reasonable and necessary.
KX: Requirements specified in the medical policy have been met.

================*FAST FACTS in a NUTSHELL*

Continued use of a Group 2 support surface is covered until the ulcer is healed or, if healing does not continue, there is documentation in the medical record to show that: (1) other aspects of the care plan are being modified to promote healing, or (2) the use of the Group 2 support surface is medically necessary for wound management. In cases for which a Group 2 product is inappropriate, a Group 1 or 3 support surface could be covered if coverage criteria for that group are met. For more information, go to Medicare's Program Integrity Manual (PIM), Chapter 3, Section 3.4.1.1, at http://www.cms.gov/manuals/downloads/pim83c03.pdf

In an effort to empower nurses across the continuum of care to order support surfaces in a timely manner for the patient, a sample Tracking Form is provided in Exhibit 15.2. Patients travel from room to room, and it is sometimes impossible to keep track of the beds. Tracking forms leave paper trails, provide documentation, and make staff aware of indications, feasibility, and cost.

Exhibit 15.2   Sample Bed Tracking Form

BED TRACKING
PT. NAME_____ROOM #_____
PT. HOSPITAL #_____PT. WT._____
DATE PLACED_____DATE REMOVED_____
ON REF#_____OFF REF#_____
BED COMPANY (EXAMPLE: HILROM)_____
PHONE NUMBER_____

Continued

Exhibit 15.2 *Continued*

□ SYNERGY AIR ELITE (SAE) Overlay with blower: 36-inch, 600 pound capacity. (COST)
(Low air loss, alternating air pressure)
*Indications: Low to moderate risk. Moisture management, incontinence and/or has skin maceration.

□ CLINITRON RITE HITE Air Fluidized Therapy: 350 pound capacity. (COST)
*Indications: High risk, multiple Stage III/IV burns, flaps, grafts, excessive maceration/draining wounds.

□ TRIFLEX II BARIATRIC BED: 1,000 pound capacity and– 37-to-48-inch width frame. (COST)
*Indications: High risk, drop-down foot rails, scale, optional trapeze, foam surface.

□ EXCELCARE BARIATRIC BED: 1,000 pound capacity and 40-to-50-inch width frame (COST)
*Indications: High risk, pressure-redistribution surface, optional low air loss, scale. With air scale/trapeze.

□ FLUIDIZED AIR–RITE HITE: Weight limit, 215 pounds.
*Indications: Same indications as Rite Hite but cannot raise the head of the bed.

BED COMPANY (EXAMPLE: SIZEWISE)_____
PHONE NUMBER_____

□ Mighty Air: 39-inch   □ Commode □ Lift □ Walker
   mattress (COST)
□ Mighty Air: 48-inch   □ Commode □ Lift □ Walker
   mattress (COST)
*Indications: Low air loss, bariatric, alternating air pressure.

□ Big Turn: 39-inch   □ Commode □ Lift □ Walker
   mattress (COST)
□ Big Turn: 48-inch   □ Commode □ Lift □ Walker
   mattress (COST)

Continued

Exhibit 15.2 *Continued*

*Indications: Low air loss, bariatric, alternating air pressure, pulmonary feature.

☐ Bariatric Sizewise Bed ☐ Commode ☐ Lift ☐ Walker (COST)
Needed with a mattress above.
Note: Has a foam mattress and scale.
*Indications: Adjustable frame and length, assist side rails, and turn-assist pressure redistribution.

HOSPITAL OWNED

ICU
☐ RENTED (COST) OR OWNED
Total Care Sports (Hill-Rom Computer): Low air loss, alternating pressure, pulmonary feature.
*Indications: Moisture management, incontinence and/or skin maceration, temperature control.

FLOORS
☐ PrimeAir (Hill-Rom Non-powered: Blue/Gray): Pressure redistribution.
*Indications: Prevention and treatment of Stages I and II pressure ulcers (non-complicated patients)

☐ VersiCare (Hill-Rom Powered: Blue with frame): Alternating pressure with heel feature.
*Indications: Reduces falls (lowest-height bed)

IV

Legal Aspects and Regulations

16

Qualifications and Certifications for Specializing in Wound Care

INTRODUCTION

So you want to be a wound care nurse? The work is hard, but the pay is (for some) better than we ever thought possible, and the career can take you all over the world, or not. Most nurses either love wound care or hate it. I happen to love it, and for those who are intrigued and fascinated with pursuing this wonderful labor of love, I have some tips. As discussed in previous chapters, wound care nursing requires knowledge of the processes of wounds, as well as appropriate judgment in care and treatment of wounds. The field of wound care management offers a variety of choices, such as hospital-based wound care, hyperbaric medicine, wound ostomy nursing, wound clinic care, and consulting. Wound care is a specialty that is diverse and shared by nurses, physicians, physical therapists, and technicians (to name a few). Certification is involved, and there are different levels of specialization. The certification process is as individual as the unique person pursuing the career.

In this chapter, you will learn:

1. About the top governing bodies in wound care and what kind of certifications these organizations offer, as well as the minimum prerequisites and fees for each program.
2. About some wound care organizations and associations.

WOUND CERTIFICATION PROGRAMS

Wound care specialization is exciting and rewarding when it is balanced with one's personal goals and career path. Various certification programs available for wound care specialization are described in the following.

Note: Fees discussed are subject to change; check the organizations' Web sites for current fee schedules.

The Wound, Ostomy, and Continence Nursing Certification Board (WOCNCB)

- *Eligibility Requirements:* Registered nurses with a BSN degree.
- *Program Includes:* A 10-week on-site program (or split-option program), 120 hours of clinical experience, and the passing of an exam after three separate courses of post-graduate study.
- *Certification Cost:* $300 plus a $50 fee for each additional specialty certification. There are additional costs for a preceptorship.
- *Certification Validity:* The Certified **Wound Care** Nurse (CWCN), Certified **Wound** and Ostomy Care Nurse (CWOCN), Certified Ostomy Care **Nurse** (COCN), Certified Continence Care **Nurse** (CCCN), and Certified **Wound** Ostomy Nurse (CWON) programs are accredited by the National Commission for Certifying Agencies (NCCA), the American Board of Nursing Specialties (ABNS), and the WOCN. Certification is valid for 5 years. Advanced practice credentialing in

wound, ostomy, and continence nursing is also available. CFCN™ is also available but not accredited.

- *Recertification Requirements:* A recertification fee is required plus a $50.00 fee for each additional specialty certification, plus examination or portfolio submission fees.
- *Contact Information:* WOCNCB, 555 E. Wells St., Suite 1100, Milwaukee, WI 53202, 888-496-2622, wocncb. org and Emory University Wound, Ostomy, and Continence Nursing Education Center (WOCNEC), Room AT732, 1365 Clifton Rd. NE, Atlanta, GA 30322-1013, 404-778-4067.

The American Academy of Wound Management (AAWM)

- *Eligibility Requirements:* At least a bachelor's degree, with a minimum of 3 years of documented experience researching wound related treatments or delivering clinical care to injured patients. Available to post-residency physicians, biomedical scientists, nurses, and qualified non-health care professionals with documented evidence of working in the wound management field.
- *Program Includes:* The program does not offer or endorse precertification training. *Certification Cost:* $550 for testing; $200 for retesting.
- *Recertification Requirements:* A $150 annual fee and six continuing education units (CEUs); a $400 recertification fee and exam every 10 years.
- *Certification Validity:* The Certified Wound Specialist (CWS) program is accredited by the National Commission for Certifying Agencies (NCCA) and the AAWM. Certification and is valid for 10 years.
- *Contact Information:* AAWM, 1155 15th Street NW, Suite 500, Washington, DC, 20005, 202-457-8408, aawm.org

The Wound Care Education Institute (WECI)

- *Eligibility Requirements:* Current employment as a physician, registered nurse, physical therapist, or physician's assistant or in a related medical field that requires the care and treatment of wounds. Also, a minimum of 2 years of' full-time or 4 years of' part-time experience is required.
- *Program Includes:* A 5-day on-site training course and the NAWC exam at the conclusion of the course.
- *Certification Cost:* The regular registration cost for individuals is $2,897.
- *Certification Validity:* The Wound Care Certification (WCC) program is accredited by the National Alliance of Wound Care Credentialing Board (NAWCCB). Certification is valid for 5 years.
- *Contact Information:* The Wound Care Education Institute, 1700 Park Street, Suite 100, Naperville, IL, 60563, 877-462-9234, wcei.net

The National Alliance of Wound Care (NAWC)

- *Eligibility Requirements:* An active, unrestricted license as a registered nurse, licensed practical/vocational nurse, nurse practitioner, physical therapist, physical therapist assistant, occupational therapist, physician, or physician's assistant. Participants also must be graduates of NAWC or have 2 years of full-time or 4 years of part-time active involvement in the field of wound care. (Visit the Web site given in the following for other options.)
- *Program Includes:* The option of a 4-week classroom program or 120 hours of clinical experience with a WCC specialist as well as an exam.
- *Certification Cost:* $330.
- *Recertification Fee and Requirements:* A fee is required as well as successful completion of one of the following: the NAWC training program, or 60 hours of continuing

education, or an examination. (Other options are available.)

- *Certification Validity:* The WCC is accredited by the National Commission for Certifying Agencies (NCCA). Certification is valid for 5 years.
- *Contact Information:* The National Alliance of Wound Care, 5464 N. Port Washington Road #134, Glendale, WI 53217, 877-WCC-NAWC (1-877-922-6292), www. nawccb.org/

Wound Care Organizations and Associations

The wound care community is vast and passionate, with members working together toward the common vision of excellence in wound management. There are too many organizations to list them all here.

═══════════════*FAST FACTS in a NUTSHELL*

Wound-Care Associations, Organizations, and Journals

Those who are interested in pursuing a wound care career may find the following Internet sites very insightful.

- *Advances in Skin and Wound Care Journal:* aswcjournal
- The Association for the Advancement of Wound Care (AAWC): www.aawconline.org
- The American Diabetes Association: www.diabetes. org
- The American Professional Wound Care Association (APWCA): www.apwca.org
- The American Academy of Wound Management (AAWM): www.aawm.org
- The American College of Hyperbaric Medicine (ACHM): www.achm.org

Continued

Continued

- *The Journal of Wound Care (JWC):* www.journalof woundcare.com
- The National Alliance of Wound Care (NAWC): www.nawccb.org
- The National Pressure Ulcer Advisory Panel (NPUAP): www.npuap.org
- Ostomy Wound Management: www.o-wm.com
- The Wound Healing Society (WHS): www.wound heal.org
- The Wound, Ostomy and Continence Nurses' Society (WOCNS): www.wocn.org
- Wound Care Education Resources: wound consultant.com
- Wounds: www.woundsresearch.com
- Worldwide Wounds: www.worldwidewounds.com

17

Awareness of Your Facility's Reputation: Certification and Accreditation

INTRODUCTION

"Mirror, mirror, on the wall, who's the fairest of them all?" When it comes to a facility's reputation, quality patient care is certainly not subjective, as is a beauty contest. In fact, facilities should be judged by their standard of quality patient care. This is measured by objective data, which is also available to the public. The wound care nurse understands the difference in measured quality care versus the subjective reputation of a facility. He or she knows all about the complex system—at its core. In the facility where he or she works, the wound care nurse is one of the creative frontline workers in the trenches, taking responsibility for and administering patient care. The wound care nurse also takes very seriously the rankings of the facility, often, for instance, playing a big role in Pressure Ulcer Prevalence and Incidence (P & I) studies.

To the wound care nurse and his or her colleagues, these empirical outcome rankings are the mirror on *the wall. Does that imply that a wound care nurse would not seek a position at a facility with low rankings? Absolutely not! A wound care nurse is passionately driven by excellence, not only providing quality care, but also striving to improve the standard of quality itself. This chapter is dedicated to helping nurses understand who provides the certification and accreditation to health care facilities and organizations. A passionate, responsible nurse wants to work in an environment where he or she is driven to excel in the highest standards of safe and effective care.*

In this chapter, you will learn:

1. About the Joint Commission, an independent, non-profit organization that accredits and certifies more than 18,000 health care facilities in the United States.
2. About the criteria for a hospital to earn Magnet Status from the American Nurses' Credentialing Center.
3. About other organizations that play a role in the standardization of medical facilities outside the hospital setting.

THE JOINT COMMISSION (JC)

Formerly known as the Joint Commission on Accreditation of Healthcare Organizations (JACHO), the Joint Commission (JC) is a not-for-profit organization that is responsible for hospital accreditation in the United States. Its certification is recognized by most state governments as a requirement of licensure. From 1951 to 2008, the JC was considered the essential body for accreditation, and its accreditation was also recognized as a requirement for health care providers to receive Medicaid and Medicare. Since that time, effective July 15, 2010, the JC's accreditation program has been under the authority of the Centers for Medicare and Medicaid (CMS).

=====*FAST FACTS in a NUTSHELL*

- All health care facilities are subject to a 3-year accreditation cycle.
- Survey findings during these 3 years are not made public, but the facility's accreditation decision is.
- Surveys are unannounced.
- A JC surveyor examines current processes, policies, standards, and procedures, and they must be in compliance with the JC.
- The facility is responsible for updating its standards and expanding patient safety goals on a yearly basis.
- This information is posted on the Internet and is available to all.
- National Patient Safety Goals (NPSGs) provide some of the critical guidelines used to promote and enforce major changes in patient safety.
- Frequently asked questions regarding JC standards are organized by specialty manuals. See http://www.jointcommission.org/Standards/FAQs/

The Joint Commission Resources (JCR) is an affiliate designated by the JC to publish materials that help improve safety and quality of health care, such as *Clinical Care Improvement Strategies Preventing Pressure Ulcers*, which can be downloaded as a PDF. Another important document listed under Patient Safety is *The Official "Do Not Use" List of Abbreviations*. Accredited organizations are required not to use these abbreviations. The JC site is http://www.jointcommission.org

THE ANCC MAGNET RECOGNITION PROGRAM

The American Nurses Credentialing Center (ANCC) is the world's largest and most prestigious nurse credentialing organization, and it is a subsidiary of the American Nurses Association (ANA). The ANCC developed The Magnet Recognition Program to recognize health care facilities that provide nursing excellence. Established in 1983 with 41 "magnet" hospitals, the AAN developed the Forces of

Magnetism, which are characteristics that seem to distinguish magnet hospitals from other hospitals. The ANCC vision for magnet hospitals is that they serve as the source "of "knowledge and expertise for the delivery of nursing care globally." These facilities are expected by the ANCC to lead the reformation of health care while sharing a common foundation of magnet principles. The new generation model for the Magnet Program has five components, which acknowledge global issues in nursing and health care.

═══════════════════════*FAST FACTS in a NUTSHELL*

The ANCC's Original 14 Forces of Magnetism

Transformational Leadership
- *Quality of Nursing Leadership (Force #1)*
- *Management Style (Force #3)*

Structural Empowerment

- *Organizational Structure (Force #2)*
- *Personnel Policies and Programs (Force #4)*
- *Community and the Health Care Organization (Force #10)*
- *Image of Nursing (Force #12)*
- *Professional Development (Force #14)*

Exemplary Professional Practice

- *Professional Models of Care (Force #5)*
- *Consultation and Resources (Force #8)*
- *Autonomy (Force #9)*
- *Nurses as Teaches (Force #11)*
- *Interdisciplinary Relationships (Force #13)*

New Knowledge, Innovations, and Improvements

- *Quality Improvement (Force #7)*

Empirical Quality Outcomes

- *Quality of Care (Force #6)*

To learn more about the ANCC and its Magnet program, go to http://www.nursecredentialing.com

Suggested reading from this site for wound care nurses includes the articles "Exemplary Professional Practice," "Nurses in Action," and "Pathway to Excellence Research References."

Outside the Hospital Arena

All external medical facility accreditation programs vary related to cost, clinical standards, skill, and ethical principles. It is important to note that accreditation methods are not the same as government-controlled initiatives. The provision and improvement of health care is constantly changing. Whatever accreditation processes that a facility or organization chooses, government-controlled initiatives oversee them. Not all medical facilities use JC accreditation.

═══════════════════════*FAST FACTS in a NUTSHELL*

Some National Accreditation Organizations Other Than the JC

- *Community Health Accreditation Program (CHAP):* Assesses community health organizations.
- *Accreditation Commission for Health Care (ACHC):* Assesses home health and hospice providers.
- *The Compliance Team:* Conducts Exemplary Provider Accreditation Programs for durable medical equipment (DME).
- *Healthcare Quality Association on Accreditation (HQAA):* Provides accreditation for home medical equipment providers.
- *DNV Healthcare:* Has been approved by the CMS to accredit hospitals and is sometimes used as an alternative to the JC.

AMERICAN MEDICAL DIRECTORS ASSOCIATION (AMDA)

The AMDA is an association made up of members from the American Medical Association (AMA) and the American Society of Internal Medicine. The mission of AMDA is to "provide education, advocacy, information, and professional development to promote the delivery of quality long term care medicine." The organization is dedicated to excellence of care for long-term care (LTC) facilities.

The AMDA's Priority Areas and Overall Goals

1. To be the premier information source on patient care for LTC facilities.
2. To encourage greater physician involvement in LTC facilities.
3. To develop initiatives.
4. To increase the knowledge base, clinical skills, and excellence of care for LTC facilities.

═══════════════════════════*FAST FACTS in a NUTSHELL*

The AMDA has a wealth of clinical tools related to LTC available for download and purchase:

Clinical Practice Guidelines: Twenty-five guidelines organized by clinical practice guideline subjects.
Audiocasts: Subjects such as insomnia, diabetes, and deep vein thrombosis.
Clinical Corners: Information, resources, links, self-studies, etc.
Forms: Admission, enteral, 24-hour, order sheets, transfers, etc.

Continued

Continued

Practitioner's Tool Box

Protocols: A guide to assist nursing staff in patient assessment and data collection prior to consulting with a physician.
Tool Kits: Help with implementation.

THE OUTCOME AND ASSESSMENT INFORMATION SET (OASIS)

For home health agencies to receive payment from Medicare, they must submit a detailed OASIS assessment report on every patient at the initial treatment visit, and every 9 weeks thereafter. Nurses must comply with OASIS standards. The majority of agency patient care (in the home health setting) is 100% covered by Medicare. CMS oversees OASIS regulations. Not adhering strictly to these regulations is detrimental to the financial viability of any agency.

FAST FACTS in a NUTSHELL

Requirements for a Patient to Qualify for Medicare Paid Home Care

1. The patient must have a physician's order for home care.
2. The patient must be homebound.
3. The patient must need skilled care.
4. The care must be intermittent, temporary, and with a realistic end point. For instance, a healing wound requires fewer visits as it heals. When the wound heals as expected, this is the realistic end point.
5. The care required must be reasonable and necessary.

The current (2010) version of OASIS is called OASIS-C. Efforts are being made to assess and measure the quality of patient care across post-acute care settings. The instrument being developed for this program is called the Continuity Assessment Record Evaluation (CARE). CARE is meant to correlate data from three well-known CMS clinical assessment instruments:

- *The Minimum Data Set (MDS)*: For nursing homes.
- *The Uniform Data Set for Medical Rehabilitation (Functional Independence Measure [FIM])*: For rehabilitation facilities.
- *OASIS:* For home care.

For information regarding OASIS-C Guidance Manual changes, go to http://www.wocn.org/pdfs/About_Us/News/Chapter1.pdf

Importance of Understanding the Accreditation and Certification Process

It is important for a wound care nurse looking for a position or already working in a facility to understand the importance of the information in this chapter. For a new wound care nurse who is applying for a position at a facility, doing some research and finding out who accredits and has certified the facility will make his or her résumé stand out among others. A positive knowledge base in this area (not necessarily at an expert level) indicates to the employer a willingness to partner with the facility to build a reputation of measurable quality care. Wound care nurses who understand the accreditation and certification process and are willing to work within them are very valuable to their facility.

18

The Centers for Medicare and Medicaid Healthcare's Common Procedure Coding System: Guidelines and Reimbursement

INTRODUCTION

Wound care nurses must understand how reimbursement works. A wound care nurse is paid either hourly or by salary for providing services, applying wound care products, and implementing wound care technology as needed. The facility is reimbursed for the care provided by the wound care nurse from The Centers for Medicare and Medicaid (CMS) and other related health insurance programs. For the CMS and other related programs to ensure that claims are processed in an orderly manner, the Healthcare Common Procedure Coding System (HCPCS) was developed. The HCPCS is a set of health care procedural codes based on the American Medical Association's Current Procedural Terminology (CPT). The HCPCS was established in 1978 to provide a standardized coding system for describing specific services and products provided in the delivery of health care. The use of these HCPCS codes, based on health care documentation, became mandatory when the Health Insurance Portability and Accountability Act of 1996 was implemented.

In this chapter, you will learn:

1. Some reimbursement requirements and guidelines based on the HCPCS.
2. Some HCPCS codes related to wound care.
3. Why the principles behind reimbursement make the wound care nurse a valuable asset to the facility.

THE TWO HCPCS LEVELS

Level I

Level I codes are maintained by the American Medical Association (AMA). These are Current Procedural Terminology (CPT-4) codes that identify medical services and procedures furnished by physicians and other health care professionals.

- These codes are identifiable as having five numeric digits.
- Debridement procedures performed primarily in out-patient settings have CPT codes from 11040 to 11044, depending upon the type of tissue that is surgically debrided.
- Active wound care management codes range from 97597 to 97602. Examples of services with these codes range from negative-pressure wound therapy to selective and non-selective debridement.

Level II

Level II codes are maintained primarily by the CMS. These codes are the standard coding system used to distinguish products, supplies, and services not included in the CPT-4 codes. Wound care related examples of these are durable medical equipment (DME), prosthetics, orthotics, and wound care supplies.

- These codes are HCPCS codes that are identifiable by a single letter and four numeric digits.
- HCPCS codes represent over 4,000 separate categories of manufacturers' products.
- Device categories, new technology procedures, drugs, biologicals, and radiopharmaceuticals fall under Level II HCPCS as Outpatient Prospective Payment System (OPPS) status indicators.
- Temporary codes are also included in Level II HCPCS:
  - *G Codes:* Used for procedures and professional services that have no CPT code.
  - *K Codes:* Temporary codes for Medicare administrative contractors that supply DME that has no CPT codes.
  - *Q and S Codes:* Temporary national codes that are non-Medicare, such as the S codes used by Blue Cross/Blue Shield Association, the private sector, and the Medicaid program.

Understanding Reimbursement Guidelines

How do these codes apply to the wound care nurse? First and foremost, they are related to patient compliance. A patient is not likely to be compliant with a treatment plan if he or she cannot even meet the deductibles or pay for the treatment. Understanding the basics of a patient's reimbursement plan will enable the wound care nurse to provide the most cost-effective and best quality of care. Nurses who show an interest in supply costs balance their care for the patient and facility that they work for. A good example is barrier creams, which range from $6.00 per tube to upwards of $175.00 per tube. What level of cream is really necessary?

=====*FAST FACTS in a NUTSHELL*

Become familiar with these reimbursement guidelines:

- What is the patient setting? Is it acute care, home health care, or a skilled nursing facility?
- Who is paying for the care? Medicare, an HMO, a health insurance provider, or Workman's Compensation?
- If an insurance provider is paying, what are the coverage benefits, deductibles, and copayments?
- Is treatment a medical necessity? Does the patient diagnosis support the medical necessity?
- Do the dressing, services, and technology support the medical necessity?
- Are the codes correctly verified by Medicare or other sources?
- What are the fees or assigned payment amounts for services?

LEVEL II HCPCS CODES FOR WOUND CARE PRODUCTS

Table 18.1 provides a list of wound care products and their codes. Note that the codes are not all inclusive for the generic categories listed.

The coding process is complex, and assignment of an HCPCS code to a product does not imply approval, endorsement, or a guarantee of a claim reimbursement for products. To learn more about the HCPCS codes and their relationship to reimbursement, go to www.cms.gov/home/medicare.asp

TABLE 18.1   Level II HCPCS Codes for Wound Care Products

Wound Care Product	HCPCS Code
Absorbent Dressings	A6234 – A6238
Abdomen Holder/Binder Pad	L1270
Adhesives	A4364
Adhesive Bandages	A6413
Adhesive Disc or Foam Pads	A5126
Adhesive Remover	A4455-A4456
Alcohol Wipes	A4245
Alginate Type Dressings	A6196-16199
Betadine	A4246-A4247
Cleanser, Wound	A6260
Collagen Wound Dressing	A6020-A6024
Composite Dressing	A6200-A6205
Compression Bandage	A4460
Compression Burn Garment	A6501-A6512
Compression Stockings	A6530-A6549
Contact Layer	A6206-A6208
Elastic Garments	A4466
Filler, Wound (Not Classified)	A6261-A6262
Film, Transparent	A6257-A6259
Foam	A6209-A6215

Continued

TABLE 18.1   Level II HCPCS Codes for Wound Care Products   *Continued*

Gauze	A6216-A6230, A6402-A6406
Gauze, Impregnated	A6222-A6233, A6266
Gauze, Non-impregnated	A6402-A6404, A6216-A6221
Hydrocolloid	A6234-A6241
Hydrogel Dressings	A6242-A6248, A6231-A6233
Iodine Swabs/Wipes	A4247
Moisturizer, Skin	A6250
Negative-Pressure Therapy Pump	E2402
Negative-Pressure Accessories	A6550
Non-contact Wound Warming Cover	E0231-E0232
Protectant, Skin Sealant, Moisturizer	A6250
Specialty Absorptive	A6251-A6256
Sterile Water	A4216-A4217, A4714
Topical Hyperbaric Oxygen Chamber	A4575
Transparent Film	A6257-A6259
Tubular Dressings	A6457

Making Cost-Effective Decisions Regarding Wound Care

A wound care nurse must understand his or her facility's reimbursement environment because the nurse plays an important role in determining what resources and supplies to use for patient care. The wound care nurse must understand strategies and responsibilities regarding how his or her decisions and actions generate costs to the facility. Making cost-effective decisions while working within the contractual constraints of the facility will help nurse advocates maximize patient resources. Remember, communicating with patients regarding the cost of their care is important. The information a patient provides will facilitate the development of a realistic treatment plan, shed light on other options, involve the patient in decision making, and increase compliance.

APPENDIX

Description of Skin Lesions

PRIMARY LESIONS – Primary lesions are physical changes in the skin considered to be caused directly by the disease process. Types of primary lesions are rarely specific to a single disease entity.

Macule – A macule is a change in the color of the skin. It is flat; if you were to close your eyes and run your fingers over the surface of a purely macular lesion, you could not detect it. A macule greater than 1 cm may be referred to as a *patch*.
Image: *Cafe-au-lait macules*

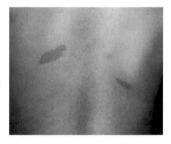

Papule – A papule is a solid raised lesion that has distinct borders and is less than 1 cm in diameter. Papules may have a variety of shapes in profile (domed, flat topped, umbilicated) and may be associated with secondary features such as crusts or scales.
Image: *Molluscum contagiosum*

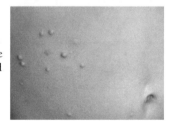

Note: With grateful appreciation to Gary Williams, MD and Murray Katcher, MD Department of Pediatrics, The University of Wisconsin, Madison. For permission to reprint "Primary Care Dermatology Module Nomenclature of Skin Lesions."

Nodule – A nodule is a raised solid lesion more than 1 cm and may be in the epidermis, dermis, or subcutaneous tissue.
Image: *Basal cell carcinoma*

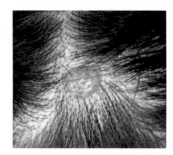

Tumor – A tumor is a solid mass of the skin or subcutaneous tissue; it is larger than a nodule. (Please bear in mind that this definition does not mean that the lesion is a neoplasm.)
Image: *Xanthomas*

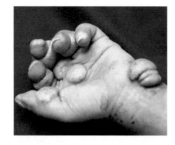

Plaque – A plaque is a solid, raised, flat-topped lesion greater than 1 cm in diameter. It is analogous to the geological formation, the plateau.
Image: *Psoriasis*

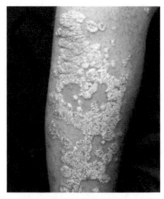

Vesicle – Vesicles are raised lesions less than 1 cm. in diameter that are filled with clear fluid. Image: *Hand/foot/mouth disease*

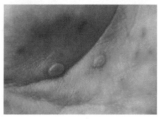

Bullae – Bullae are circumscribed, fluid-filled lesions that are greater than 1 cm. (Note the differences between bullae and vesicles)
Image: *Stevens-Johnson syndrome*

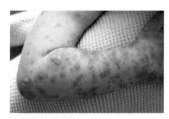

Pustule – Pustules are circumscribed, elevated lesions that contain pus. They are most commonly infected (as in folliculitis) but may be sterile (as in pustular psoriasis)
Image: Group A beta-hemolytic streptococcus infection

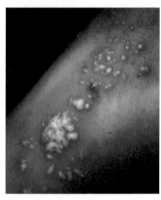

Wheal – A wheal is an area of edema in the upper epidermis.
Image: Urticaria (or hives) on back

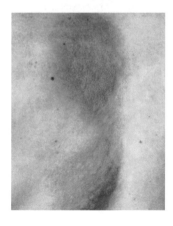

Burrow – Burrows are linear lesions produced by infestation of the skin and formation of tunnels (e.g., with infestation by the scabitic mite or by cutaneous larva migrans).
Image: *Cutaneous larva migrans*

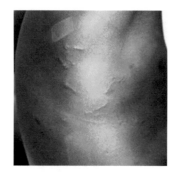

Telangiectasia – Telangiectasia are the permanent dilatation of superficial blood vessels in the skin and may occur as isolated phenomena or as part of a generalized disorder, such as ataxia telangiectasia.
Image: Spider or starburst telangiectasia

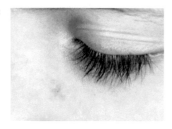

SECONDARY LESIONS – Secondary lesions may evolve from primary lesions, or may be caused by external forces such as scratching, trauma, infection, or the healing process. The distinction between a primary and secondary lesion is not always clear.

Scale – Secondary lesions may evolve from primary lesions, or may be caused by external forces such as scratching, trauma, infection, or the healing process. The distinction between a primary and secondary lesion is not always clear.
Notice *the papules in the center of the photo.* Image: *Cutaneous fungal infection*

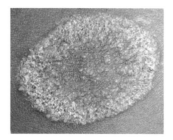

Crust – Crusting is the result of the drying of plasma or exudate on the skin. Remember that crusting is different from scaling. The two terms refer to different phenomena and are not interchangeable. One can usually be distinguished from the other by appearance alone. Image: *Impetigo*

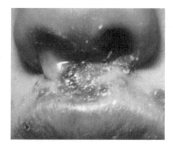

Atrophy – Atrophy is the thinning or absence of the epidermis or subcutaneous fat.
Notice the thinning or absence of the epidermis or subcutaneous fat (striae) secondary to chronic systemic steroid administration. Image: *Striae areas*

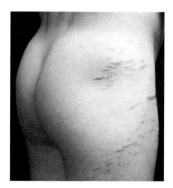

Lichenification – Lichenification refers to a thickening of the epidermis seen with exaggeration of normal skin lines. It is usually due to chronic rubbing or scratching of an area. Image: *Pruritic scabies*

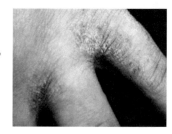

Erosion – Erosions are slightly depressed areas of skin in which part or all of the epidermis has been lost.
Image: *Chemical burn*

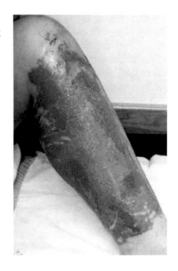

Excoriation – Excoriation is traumatized or abraded skin caused by scratching or rubbing.
Image: *Swimmers' itch*

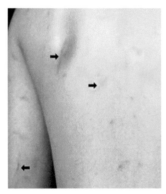

Fissure – A fissure is linear cleavage of skin that extends into the dermis.
Image: *Fissure in palm of hand*

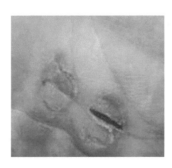

Ulceration – Ulcerations occur when there is necrosis of the epidermis and dermis and sometimes of the underlying subcutaneous tissue. Image: *Electrical burn*

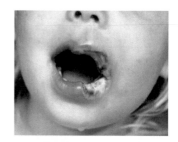

Scar – Scars are the permanent fibrotic changes that occur on the skin following damage to the dermis. Scars may have secondary pigment characteristics. Image: *Intravenous infiltrate*

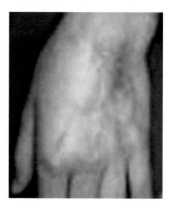

Eschar – An eschar is a hard plaque covering an ulcer implying extensive tissue necrosis, infarcts, deep burns, or gangrene. Image: *Meningococcemia*

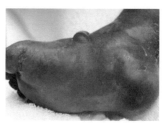

Keloids – Keloids are an exaggerated connective tissue response of injured skin that extend beyond the edges of the original wound. Image: *Lymph node biopsy site*

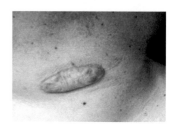

Petechiae, Purpura, and Ecchmoses –
Three terms that refer to bleeding
that occurs in the skin are petechiae,
purpura, and ecchymoses. Generally,
the term "petechiae" refers to smaller
lesions. "Purpura" and "ecchymoses"
are terms that refer to larger lesions.
In certain situations purpura may be
palpable. In all situations, petechiae,
ecchymoses, and purpura do not
blanch when pressed.
Image: *Henoch-Schönlein Purpura*

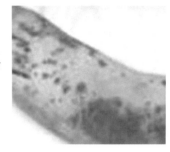

PATTERNS AND DISTRIBUTION – Not only is the appearance of
lesions important, but the pattern and distribution on the skin is as
well.

Annular – Annular lesions are seen
in a ring shape. Tinea corporis,
erythema migrans (the lesion
associated with Lyme disease), and
granuloma annulare are three
common examples. Image: *Tinea
corporis*

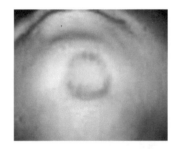

Discrete – Discrete lesions tend to
remain separate. This is a helpful
descriptive term but has little specific
diagnostic significance.
Notice that the lesions are vesicles.
Image: *Varicella in discrete pattern*

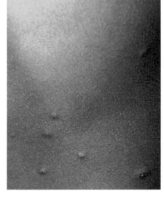

Clustered – Clustered lesions are those that are grouped together. They are commonly seen in herpes simplex or with insect bites, for example. Image: *Herpes simplex*

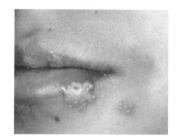

Confluent – Confluent lesions tend to run together.
Notice that the macular lesions have become confluent. Image: *Kawasaki's disease*

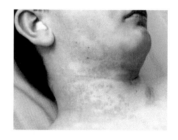

Dermatomal, Zosteriform – Dermatomal, zosteriform lesions follow a dermatome. The lesions of varicella zoster (also known as shingles) are the classic example, but there are other lesions that may assume the same pattern. Image: *Varicella zoster*

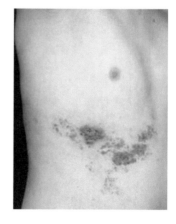

Eczematoid – Eczematoid lesions are inflamed with a tendency toward clustering, oozing, or crusting.
Image: *Atopic dermatitis*

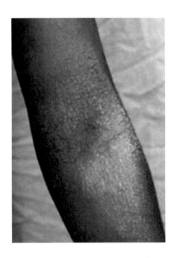

Follicular – It is sometimes helpful to determine if lesions specifically involve the hair follicle.
Notice the pustule lesions.
Image: *Folliculitis*

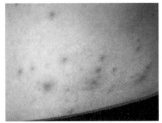

Guttate – Guttate lesions look as though someone took a dropper and dropped this lesion on the skin. Guttate lesions are characteristic of one form of psoriasis, though that is not the only example.
Image: *Guttate psoriasis*

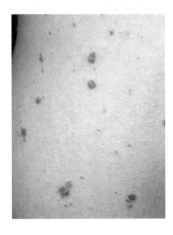

Iris or Target Lesions – Iris lesions are also known as target lesions and are a series of concentric rings. These have a dark or blistered center. These lesions are frequently seen with erythema multiforme but not exclusively so.
Image: *Kawasaki's disease*

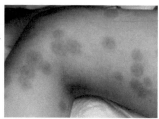

Koebner Phenomenon – The Koebner phenomenon, also called the isomorphic response, refers to the appearance of lesions along a site of injury. This phenomenon is seen in a variety of conditions; for example, lichen planus, warts, molluscum contagiosum, psoriasis, lichen nitidus, and the systemic form of juvenile rheumatoid arthritis. *Note the salmon colored rash where scratched.*
Image: *Juvenile rheumatoid arthritis*

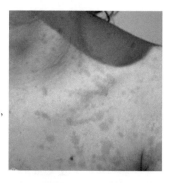

Linear Lesions – Linear lesions occur in a linear or band-like configuration. This descriptive term may apply to a wide variety of disorders. (One should be certain that the lesions are not following a dermatome.)
Image: *Lymphangitis*

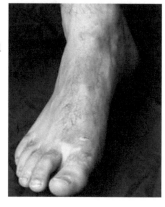

Multiform – Patients with multiform lesions have lesions of a variety of shapes.
Note the paradigm of conditions with multiform lesions: target lesions, urticarial lesions, and annular lesions.
Image: *Erythema multiforme*

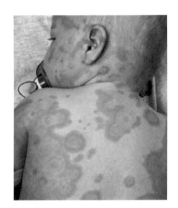

Reticular – Reticular or net-like lesions can be seen in a variety of circumstances; for example, they are very common in newborns (or even grown children and adults) as cutis marmorata or with livedo reticularis. The former fades as the skin is warmed; the latter becomes more florid. Image: *Cutis marmorata*

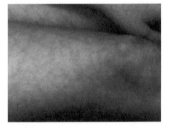

Serpiginous – Serpiginous lesions wander as though following the track of a snake. Image: *Urticaria*

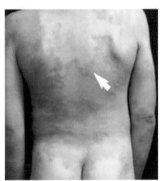

Universalis – Universalis refers to a widespread disorder that affects the entire skin.
Image: *Alopecia universalis*

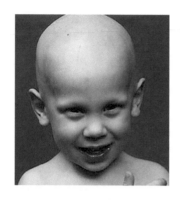

Scarlatiniform – Scarlatiniform rashes have the pattern of scarlet fever. The patient with a scarlatiniform rash has innumerable small red papules that are widely and diffusely distributed. Note that the term scarlatiniform does not mean that the patient has scarlet fever, although by definition all patients with scarlet fever have a scarlatiniform rash. Patients with a variety of other conditions such as Kawasaki's disease, viral infections, or drug reactions may have rashes with the same pattern.
Note the pinpoint papules associated with scarlet fever. Image: *Scarlet fever*

Morbilliform – The term "morbilliform" means that the patient has a rash that looks like measles. Patients with measles will have the rash but patients with Kawasaki's disease, drug reactions, or other conditions may also have a morbilliform rash. The rash consists of macular lesions that are red and are usually 2–10 mm in diameter but may be confluent in places. Image: *Measles*

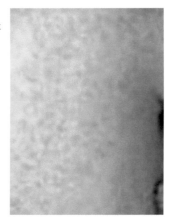

Satellite Lesions – The term is commonly used to describe a portion of the rash of cutaneous candidiasis in which a beefy red plaque may be found surrounded by numerous, smaller red macules located adjacent to the body of the main lesions. Image: *Candidal diaper dermatitis*

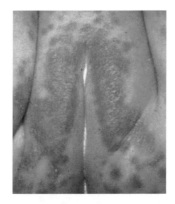

Patterns of Intentional or Unintentional Injury – One important category of skin lesions involves the form that skin lesions may take in cases of child abuse or other intentional injury (bite marks, slap marks, strap marks, burns, etc.) or in cases of unintentional injury. Abrasions are traumatically caused erosions Image: Cigarette burn

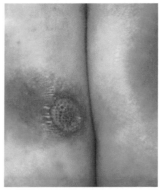

Glossary

Angiogenesis – The formation of new blood vessels from the pre-existing, surrounding blood supply. This happens during the proliferation of granulation tissue.

Asymptomatic – A person who has a disease, shows no symptoms, but can transmit it to others.

Blanching Erythema – An area of reddened tissue that turns white when pressed with the fingertip (termed blanching). This is an early indication of pressure, – not deep tissue, damage. It resolves once the fingertip is removed.

BUN – Abbreviation for blood urea nitrogen.

Dehiscence - Surgical complication where the incision opens.

Dehydration – Excessive loss of water from body tissues.

Demarcation – The line of separation between viable and non-viable tissue.

Dirty Wound – A wound that has slough or eschar present, but does not have cellulitis.

DRG - Diagnosis Related Groups (DRG) is the system for classifying hospital cases into levels reflecting hospital resource utilization.

Duration of Pressure – The evidence of low-intensity pressure over a long period of time can create tissue damage, just as high-intensity pressure can cause damage over a short period of time.

Epidermolysis – Epidermis separation and sloughing from the dermis related to collagen anchor damage between the epidermis and dermis.

Epithelium – Regeneration and migration of pink, dry, flat, and shiny epidermis across the wound surface.

Erosion – Involves partial loss of epidermis but does not extend below the epidermis. Healing occurs without scarring.

Erythema Multiform – a skin condition caused by a Type IV hypersensitivity reaction to an infection (caused by herpes simplex), or allergic reaction in response to medications. Starts and spreads quickly. Has central lesions surrounded by pale red rings called "bulls-eye"; usually symmetrical; usually affects trunk, limbs, face, and eyes.

Eschar – Thick, leathery, black, or gray devitalized (dead) tissue.

Evisceration – The abdominal organs protrude or come out from a dehisced wound.

Fibroblast – Most important cell in the production of the dermal matrix; responsible for synthesis of collagen and connective tissue.

Fluctuance – An indication of pus in a wound. The skin gets red over the lesion and when touched, it feels soft and boggy. This boggy feeling is called fluctuant.

Friction – When the skin rubs across a surface; an example is a sheet burn when a patient is pulled across the bed or when a patient is restless.

GPO – A group purchasing organization (GPO) is an entity that helps health care providers – such as hospitals, nursing homes, and home health agencies – realize savings and efficiencies by aggregating purchasing volume and using that leverage to negotiate discounts with manufacturers, distributors, and other vendors (HIGPA, 2010).

Granulation – Red, beefy, moist looking (like clusters of grapes or beads), consisting of new capillaries and connective tissue.

Growth Factors – Polypeptides that control growth and differentiation of cells.

HCPCS Code – (Often pronounced "hickpicks") Stands for the Healthcare Common ProcedureCoding System. It was established in 1978 as a way to standardize identification of medical services, supplies, and equipment. The CMS has the authority to assign HCPCS codes. Medicare and Medicaid are required to use them, but simply having a HCPCS code does not' mean

Medicare or Medicaid covers the cost of the procedure. Also, assigned HCPCS codes are not product specific.

Hemostasis – Blood clots by a protiolytic cascade that converts fibrinogen into fibrin. Fibrin becomes a web that traps red blood cells and platelets. A tampon (clot) is formed stopping the bleeding. Blood clotting induces platelet degranulation, which releases growth factors (PDGF, EGF, IGF, and TGF).

Hyperpigmented – Patches of skin that become darker

Hypertrophic – Enlargement or overgrowth of tissue related to increase in size of cells (not increase in number).

ICD-9-CM – International Classification of Diseases, 9th Revision, Clinical Modification is the official system of assigning codes to diagnoses and procedures associated with hospital utilization in the United States.

Incidence – The number (value) of new diagnosis specific cases during a certain time frame. Example: Hospital X had a total of 200 meningitis cases last year.

Intensity of Pressure – The intensity of pressure being applied externally to the skin. Example: Because of a person's inability to recognize or respond to sensation, that person may sit so long that damage to capillaries results, thus causes tissue hypoxia.

Keratinocytes – Tough, fibrous, insoluble proteins found in the basal layer, continue through differentiation until they flake off as old skin. They are resistant to changes in temperature, pH, or chemical digestion by enzymes.

Langerhan Cells – Immune cells within the epidermis that provide antigens to T lymphocytes. Low levels of Langerhan cells may lead to skin cancer and infections of the skin.

Leukocytes – White blood cells used in the inflammatory phase (also called granulocytes). They up-regulate the expression of important intracellular adhesion molecules that mediate cell-to-cell bindings.

Lipodermatosclerosis – A tapering of the legs right above the ankles with brownish-red pigmentation, pain, and induration. Think of an inverted coke bottle.

Macrophages – Monocytes that become phagocytic are referred to as macrophages. Macrophages regulate the wound healing repair process; a wound cannot' heal without them. Macrophages phagocytize bacteria, ingest dead neutrophils, synthesize nitric oxide, and produce growth factors.

Mast Cells – Found in the dermis and subcutaneous and connective tissue. They contain histamine and are the primary effector cells in an allergic reaction. They also protect against parasites, activate/proliferate eosinophils, and stimulate chemotaxis.

Melanocytes – Located in the stratum basale layer of skin and responsible for skin pigmentation. These differ in size between lighter and darker skinned people.

MS-DRG – Medicare Severity Diagnosis Related Groups, an advanced version of the origional DRG that takes into account how ill the patient is. Patients with this classification would be reimbursed at a higher rate unless the condition is a HAC.

MSDS Sheet – Material Safety Data Sheet provides both workers and emergency personnel with the proper procedures for handling or working with a particular substance (health effects, reactivity, disposal, spill/leak procedures, etc.).

Myofibroblast – The most numerous cells in mature granulation tissue. They are aligned within the wound along the lines of contraction. Think of fibroblasts as "transformers" that turn into myofibroblasts, which connect with EMC to contract the wound.

Neoplasia – An abnormal mass or new growth of abnormal cells (tumor).

Osmosis – The movement of (water) through a semipermeable membrane, from lower solute concentration to high solute concentration.

pH – A slightly acidic pH helps prevent bacterial penetration or colonization (4.2 to 5.6). Normal pH of the blood is slightly neutral (7.4). A significant acidic or alkaline change can have health effects such as lowered perfusion, arrhythmia, and hypoventilation. Dressing materials and adhesives can change wound fluid pH. A lower pH (such as acetic acid – 2.4) is an effective antiseptic in controlling bacteria; however, it may be toxic to fibroblasts.

Perfusion Function – Assessment of blood perfusion through the microvascular network (Doppler is a tool used to monitor perfusion function).

Prevalence – A measurement (ratio) of the frequency of a particular condition at a specific point in time. Example: The ER unit treated 100 people last month; 10 had pressure ulcers, so 10% had pressure ulcers).

Pressure Ulcer Risk Assessment Tools – Examples are the Braden Scale, Gosnell Scale, Knoll Scale, Norton Scale, or Waterlow Scale.

Purulent Drainage – Drainage consisting of pus usually with offensive odor.

Pyrexia - Fever

Risk Factor – A hazard that makes a person vulnerable to disease or infection such as smoking.

Sanguineous Drainage – Bright red (considered new or fresh) bleeding.

Sensitivity – Measures the percentage of patients who did develop pressure-related injuries and were identified as being at risk.

Serosanguineous Drainage – Serous fluid mixed with blood; clear, pink, and watery.

Serous Drainage – Clear, pale yellow or amber, thin, watery fluid.

Shear – When the skin is held in place but the skeleton pulls (via gravity) the body down. Shear and pressure cause undermining in the deep tissues. Example: When the head of the bed is elevated greater then 30 degrees and the patient slides down.

Skin Buds – New epitithelial granulation made of small nodules that look like goosebumps.

Slough – White, or yellow, loose, stringy fibrin, necrotic tissue.

Specificity – Measures the percentage of patients who did not develop pressure-related injuries and were identified as being not at risk.

Stevens-Johnson Syndrome (SJS) – A milder form of toxic epidermal necrolysis (TEN). The rash first appears as round lesions about an inch across on the face, limbs, and soles of the feet.

TBSA – Total body surface area; a term used in burn care to calculate amount of burn area on the body. Methods include the Lund and Bower chart (considered most accurate), Rule of Nines, Palm method, Harris-Benedict formula.

Tissue Interface Pressure – An indirect quantification measurement of pressure being exerted on a capillary.

Toxic Epidermal Necrolysis (TEN) – A syndrome and life-threatening condition affecting the skin in which cell death causes the epidermis to separate from the dermis. Causes may be idiopathic or medication induced

Ulcers – Involve loss of epidermis and dermis. Healing occurs by scar formation.

Viral Shedding – Reproduction to host-cell infection, spreading from a cell, or from one part of the body to another, or from the host to other bodies.

References and
Additional Readings

ABA (2007). *American Burn Association Fact Sheet*. Retrieved July 28, 2010 from http://www.ameriburn.org/resources_factsheet. php

AHCPR Panel for the Prediction and Prevention of Pressure Ulcers in Adults (1992). *Pressure Ulcers in Adults: Prediction and Prevention*. Retrieved July 22, 2010 from http://www.ncbi.nlm. nih.gov/bookshelf/br.fcgi?book=hsahcpr&part=A9026

AHRQ (Agency for Healthcare Research and Quality) (2006). *Number of Hospital Patients with Pressure Sores Increasing*. Retrieved July 15, 2010 from http://www.ahrq.gov/news/nn/ nn041806.htm

Alvarez, O. (1988). Moist environment for healing: matching the dressing to the wound, *Ostomy Wound Management*, 21:64.

American Diabetes Association (2010). *Foot Complications*. Retrieved July 23, 2010 from http://www.diabetes.org/living- with-diabetes/complications/foot-complications.html

American Pain Society (1995). *Pain: The Fifth Vital Sign*. Retrieved from www.ampainsoc.org/advocacy/fifth.htm.

AOCD—American Osteopathic College of Dermatology (1995). *Keloids and Hypertrophic Scars*. Retrieved May 13, 2010 from www.aocd.org/skin/dermatologic_diseases/keloids/

APWCA—American Professional Wound Care Association (2010). *Proposed APWCA Photographic Guidelines for Wounds*. Retrieved from http://www.apwca.org/guidelines/photographic.cfm

Armstrong, D. and Rothenberg, G. (2002). *Maggot Therapy: Is It Viable In Wound Care?* Retrieved May 27, 2010 from http://www.podiatrytoday.com/article/895.

Baranoski, S. and Ayello, E. (2004). *Wound Care Essentials, Practice Principles.* Springhouse, PA: Lippincott Williams & Wilkins.

Bartsch, R. and Weiss, G., (2007). *Crucial Aspects of Smoking in Wound Healing after Breast Reduction Surgery.* Retrieved May 17, 2010 from http://www.surgery.upmc.edu/psjc/PDFs/10_22_08_JC_article_2_Bartsch.pdf

Battersby, L. (2009). *Best Practice in the Management of Skin Tears in Older People.* Retrieved from http://www.nursingtimes.net/nursing-practice-clinical-research/specialists/wound-care/exploring-best-practice-in-the-management-of-skin-tears-in-older-people/5000502.article

Bowler, P. (2010). *Bacterial Growth Guideline: Reassessing Its Clinical Relevance in Wound Healing.* Retrieved May17, 2010 from http://www.o-wm.com/article/1211.

Broderick, N. (2009). *Understanding Chronic Wound Healing.* Retrieved May 17, 2010 from http://www.nursingcenter.com/library/JournalArticle.asp?Article_ID=935535

Bryant, R (2001). *Acute and Chronic Wounds, Nursing Management* (2nd ed.). St. Louis, MO: Mosby, Inc.

CDC (2005). *Cutaneous Radiation Injury (CRI).* Retrieved July 26, 2010 from http://www.bt.cdc.gov/radiation/criphysicianfactsheet.asp

CDC (2009). *U.S. Obesity Trends.* Retrieved September 8, 2010 from http://www.cdc.gov/obesity/data/trends.html

CMS (2009). *Pressure Reducing Support Surfaces—Group 1 (L5067).* Retrieved September 8, 2010 from http://www.medicarenhic.com/dme/medical_review/mr_lcds/mr_lcd_current/L5067_2009-12-01_PA_2009-12.pdf

CMS (2010). *LCD for Pressure Reducing Support Surfaces—Group 2.* Retrieved September 8, 2010 from http://www.ngsmedicare.com/content.aspx?docid=21678

CMS—Centers for Medicare and Medicaid Services (2010). *HCPCS—General Information.* Retrieved May 6, 2010, from http://www.cms.gov/medhcpcsgeninfo/01 overview.asp?

CMS—Centers for Medicare and Medicaid Services (2010). Retrieved from http://search.cms.hhs.gov/search?q=wound+care+nurses

CMS MLN Matters® (2010). *Medicare Policy Regarding Pressure Reducing Support Surfaces.* Retrieved September 6, 2010 from http://www.cms.gov/manuals/downloads/pim83c03.pdf), Section 3.4.1.1

Dillon, P., Kerry Keefer, B., Blackburn, J., Houghton, P. and Krummel, T. (1993). *The Extracellular Matrix of the Fetal Wound: Hyaluronic Acid Controls Lymphocyte Adhesion.* Retrieved May 13, 2010 from http://www.oc.lm.ehu.es/

Dorner, B. (2009). *Clinical questions: fluids/hydration.* Retrieved May 10, 2010 from http://www.beckydorner.com/clinicalquestions

Elango, R., Humayun, M., Ball, R. and Pencharz, P. (2010). Evidence that protein requirements have been significantly underestimated. *Current Opinion in Clinical Nutrition & Metabolic Care,* **13**(1), 52–57.

FDA—U.S. Food and Drug Administration (2010). *Regulatory Information, (h) The Term "Device."* Retrieved May 6, 2010 from http://www.fda.gov/

Fife, K. (2007). *Pathophysiology and Epidemiology of Herpes Simplex Virus Infection.* Retrieved August 2, 2010 from http://cme.medscape.com/viewarticle/567260

Fishman, T. (2010). *Phases of Wound Healing.* Retrieved May 13, 2010 from http://medicaledu.com/phases.htm

Flanagan, M. (2010). *Improving Accuracy of Wound Measurement in Clinical Practice.* Retrieved May 24, 2010 from http://www.o-wm.com/article/2121

Fleck, C. (2007). *FAQs: Preventing and Treating Skin Tears.* Retrieved from http://www.nursingcenter.com/library/static.asp?pageid=727851

Gardner, S., Frantz, R., Saltzman, C., Hillis, S., Park, H. and Scherubel, M. (2006). *Diagnostic Validity of Quantitative Microbial Swab Techniques.* Retrieved May 17, 2010 from http://medscape.com/viewarticle/562855_2

Garra, G. and Stellke, J. (2010). *Toxic Epidermal Necrolysis.* Retrieved July 28, 2010 from http://emedicine.medscape.com/article/787323-overview

Gordon M. and Goodwin, C. (1997). Burn management: initial assessment, management, and stabilization. *Nursing Clinics of North America,* **32**(2), 297.

Halloran, D., Blume, P., Palladino, M. and Sumpio, B. (2007). *How To Perform A Thorough Vascular Exam.* Retrieved from http://www.podiatrytoday.com/article/7074.

Harris, J. and Benedict, F. (1919). *A Biometric Study of Basal Metabolism in Man*. Washington DC, Carnegie Institution of Washington. Retrieved May 11, 2010 from http://books.google.com/books

Haycock, C., Laser, C., Keuth, J., Montefour, K., Wilson, M., Austin, K. Coulen, C. and Boyle, D. (2005). Implementing evidence-based practice findings to decrease postoperative sternal wound infections following open heart surgery. *Journal of Cardiovascular Nursing*, 20(5), 299–305. Retrieved May 14, 2010 from ww.nursingcenter.com/library/JournalArticle.asp?Article_ID=599757

Heggers, J., Sazy, J., Stenberg, B., Strock, L., McCauley, R., Herndon, D. and Robson, M. (1991 Lindberg Award). *Bactericidal and Wound-Healing Properties of Sodium Hypochlorite Solutions.* Retrieved May 27, 2010 from http://journals.lww.com/burncareresearch/Abstract/1991/

Hettiaratchy, S., Moloney, D. and Clark, J. (2001). *Patients with Acute Skin Loss: Are They Best Managed on a Burns Unit?* Retrieved August 2, 2010 from http://www.ncbi.nlm.nih.gov/pmc/articles/PMC2503562/pdf/annrcse01629-0034.pdf

HIGPA—Health Industry Group Purchasing Association (2010). *What is a GPO?* Retrieved May 5, 2010 from http://www.higpa.org/

Krasner, D., Rodeheaver, G. and Sibbald, G. (2001). *Chronic Wound Care: A Clinical Source Book for Healthcare Proessionals* (3nd ed.). Wayne, PA: Mosby, HMP Communications.

McCaffery, M. and Beebe, A. (1989). *Pain: A Clinical Manual for Nursing Practice*. St. Louis: Mosby-Year Book, Inc.

Motta, G. (2010). *Wound Care Product Reimbursement: A Guide to HCPCS*. Retrieved September 21, 2010 from http://www.woundsource.com/article/product-and-technology-reimbursement-a-guide-hcpcs

NPUAP (1995). *NPUAP Statement on Reverse Staging of Pressure Ulcers.* Retrieved July 19, 1995 from http://www.npuap.org/archive/positn2.htm. "Reproduction of the National Pressure Ulcer Advisory Panel (NPUAP) materials in this document does not imply endorsement by the NPUAP of any products, organizations, companies, or any statements made by any organization or company."

NPUAP (2007). *National Pressure Ulcer Advisory Panel Support Surface Standards Initiative*. Retrieved September 6, 2010 from http://www.npuap.org/NPUAP_S3I_TD.pdf

NPUAP—National Pressure Ulcer Advisory Panel (2007). *Updated Staging System*. Retrieved May 25, 2010 from http://www.npuap.org/resources.htm.

Ovington, L. (2002). *Hanging Wet-to-Dry Dressings Out to Dry*. Retrieved May 27, 2010 from http://www.deconsolidatenow.org/Documents/9_Ovington_Article.pdf.

Payne, R. and Martin, M. (1993). *Defining and Classifying Skin Tears: Need for a Common Language*. Retrieved from http://www.ncbi.nlm.nih.gov/pubmed/8397703.

Pediani, R. (2001). *What Has Pain Relief To Do with Acute Surgical Wound Healing?* Retrieved May 4, 2010 from http://worldwide-wouds.com/2001/march/Pediani/Pain-relief-surgical-wounds.html

Porter, SE. (2001). The musculoskeletal effects of smoking. *Academy of Orthopaedic Surgeons, 9*, 9–17.

Ratiff, C. and Bryant, D. (2010). *Guideline for Prevention and Management of Pressure Ulcers*.WOCN Clinical Practice Guideline Series Number 2. Wound, Ostomy and Continence Nurses Society. Retrieved from http://www.wocn.org/About_Us/News/61/

Roget, P. (1904, Revised printing (1992). *Roget's International Thesaurus* (5th ed.). New York, NY: HarperCollins.

Ross, D. (2003). *The ABCs of Coding-for Electrical Stimulation*. Retrieved August 17, 2010 from http://www.hcpro.com/RHB-34131–882/The-ABCs-of-codingfor-electrical-stimulation.html

Russo, A., Elixhauser, A. and Healthcare Cost and Utilization Project (H-CUP) (2003). *Hospitalizations Related to Pressure Sores, 2003*. Retrieved July 15, 2010 from http://www.hcup-us.ahrq.gov/reports/statbriefs/sb3.pdf

Schultz, G. and Mast, B. (1999). *Molecular Analysis of the Environments of Healing and Chronic Wounds: Cytokines, Proteases and Growth Factors*. Retrieved May 13, 2010 from www.awma.com.au/journal/library/0701_01.pdf

Schwartz, R. and Kaplla, R. (2010). *Necrotizing Fascitis*. Retrieved July 27, 2010 from http://emedicine.medscape.com/article/1054438-overview

Speri-Hillen, J. and O'Connor, J. (2005). *Factors Driving Diabetes Care Improvement in a Large Medical Group—10 Years of Progress*. Retrieve July 22, 2010 from the AJMC at http://www.ajmc.com/supplement/managed-care/2005/2005-08-vol11-n5Suppl/Aug05-2115pS177-S185.

Stephens, D. and Bisno, A. (2005). *Practice Guidelines for the Diagnosis and Management of Skin and Soft Tissue Infections.* Retrieved July 27, 2010 from http://www.guideline.gov/summary/summary.aspx?doc_id=8206&nbr=004581&string=Necrotizing+AND+fasciitis

Straube, D. (2008). *HCPCS Codes: Frequently Asked Questions.* Retrieved May 6, 2010 from http://www.nls.org/av/FAQ's%20HCPCS.pdf

Sussman, C. (2001). Gaithersburg, Maryland. *Electrical Stimulation for Wound Healing, Wound Care Collaborative Practice Manual for Physical Therapist and Nurses* (2nd ed.). Aspen Publishers.

Suzuki, K. and Cowan, L. (2009). *Current Concepts In Wound Debridement.* Retrieved May 25, 2010 from http://www.podiatrytoday.com/current-concepts-in-wound-debridement.

Titmuss, R. (1974). *Social Policy.* Retrieved August 4, 2010 from http://books.google.com/books?id

Turnbull, G (2009). From proposal to patient: how CMS makes coverage decisions. *OWM,* **48**(4).

Wagner, F. (1981). The dysvascular foot: a system for diagnosis and treatment. *Foot Ankle,* **2**:64–122.

White, P. (2010). *Legislative: Searching for Health Policy Information on the Internet: An Essential Advocacy Skill.* Retrieved August 4, 2010 from http://www.nursingworld.org/MainMenuCategories/ANAMarketplace/ANAPeriodicals/OJIN/Columns/Legislative/Health-Policy-Information-on-the-Internet.aspx

Wood, B., Molnar, J. and Kiman, C. (2010). *Skin, Graphs.* Retrieved July 29, 2010 from http://emedicine.medscape.com/article/1295109-overview

World Health Organization (2010). *WHO's Pain Ladder.* Retrieved May 21, 2010 from http://www.who.int/cancer/palliative/painladder/en/

Wright, S. (2009). *Vulnerabilities in Medicare Payments for Pressure Reducing Support Surfaces, OEI-02-07-00421.* Retrieved September 6, 2010 from http://oig.hhs.gov/oei/reports/oei-02-07-00421.pdf

Wu, S. (2010). *Taking A Closer Look At The Impact Of Wound Bioburden.* Retrieved May 18, 2010 from http://www.podiatrytoday.com/

Index

277

Forthcoming

Printed in the United States
By Bookmasters